NORTH CAROLINA
STATE BOARD OF COMMUNITY COLLEGES
LIBRARIES
NASH TECHNICAL COLLEGE

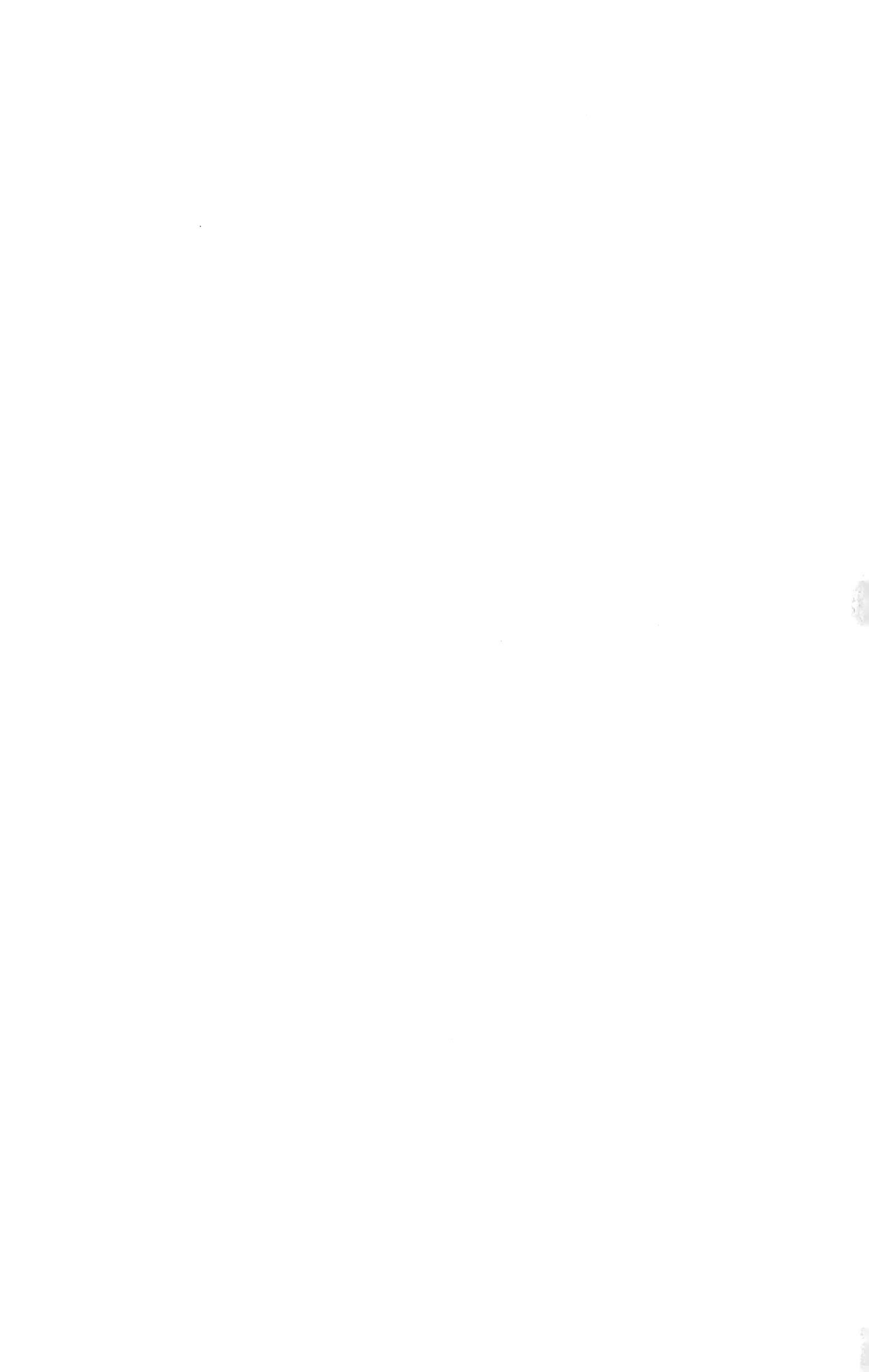

# Exercises for the Elderly

# Exercises for the Elderly

## Robert H. Jamieson

1982
Emerson Books, Inc.
Verplanck, New York 10596

*Second Printing*, 1982

©Robert H. Jamieson 1982
All rights reserved. No part of this publication may be reproduced, stored in a retrieval system, or transmitted in any form or by any means, electronic, mechanical, photocopying, recording or otherwise, without prior permission.

Published by Emerson Books, Inc. 1982
Library of Congress Catalog Card Number 81-71216
ISBN 87523-198-5

PRINTED IN 18 POINT TIMES ROMAN TYPE

# Acknowledgements

From an idea comes an outline; this is filled in and becomes a series of chapters; at this time the final touches are applied and one has a book. In my case these "final touches" came in the form of people who gave of their abilities, talent and time. I'm deeply grateful for the quality of their abilities and talents.

Mrs. Emma Haggard provided her skill with a camera to photograph the exercises; Manuel Alva, a deaf art student at Pasadena City College in Pasadena, Calif.,created the "older couple" in the last chapter; Vernon C. Dargan, age 87, and Jeanette L. Heegel, age 81, the two models who could not have been more agreeable and cooperative. I must not forget to mention Mrs. Mary Alva, Manuel's mother, who was very patient with me. Last but not least is my technical advisor, Marina Brown, who is a licensed physical therapist, who lent her expertise to smooth out the rough edges and fill in the holes; she also had the last say-so from a professional point of view. I would, also, like to mention the long suffering and gentle handling I received from my managing editor, Barry Feiden.

Bob Jamieson<br>Covina, CA.

# The Models

Vernon C. Dargan, 87 years old, exercises each morning and walks up to three miles a day. At the age of 74, he retired from Gulf Insurance Co., where he was vice president. For 20 years he worked in the reserve division of the Los Angeles County Sheriff's Department. He has a son and three grandchildren.

Jeannette L. Heegel is 81 years old. She, too, exercises each morning and walks at least one mile a day. She has two children, six grandchildren and four great grandchildren.

Both attribute their continued good health to consistent exercise and social activities.

# Table Of Contents

**Introduction**

**Preface**

1  Getting Started ............ 19
2  The Basic Exercise Program .. 35
3  A Few Wheelchair Exercises .. 73
4  Exercise Tools and Special Exercises ................. 81
5  Exercises For The Bedridden . 97
6  Isometric Exercises ......... 105
7  Starting Your Class ........ 115
8  Taking Care Of Your Back .. 135
9  Rules To Live By .......... 155

# Introduction

*Generally speaking, all parts of the body which have a function, if used in moderation, and exercise in labors to which each is accustomed, become thereby healthy and well developed and age slowly; but if unused and left idle, they become liable to disease, defective in growth and age quickly.*

Hippocrates, circa 400 B.C.

As a teacher of exercise classes in retirement homes, as well as an exercise enthusiast himself, Bob Jamieson has seen first hand the need for a book such as this. When first beginning to organize these classes, he noticed a surprising lack of reference material. He promptly decided to help correct the situation and with much dedication wrote *Exercises For The Elderly*.

As a physical therapist, I am very pleased and excited to take part in this project and also to see an exercise book such as this become available to the public. I believe it will fulfill a need that has been felt by individuals and groups alike.

With its clear instructions and illustrations, these exercises are easily understood and performed. They are of mild to moderate difficulty and therefore, in their beginning stages, make little demand on the cardiovascular and musculoskeletal systems. With increased repetitions and added resistance, however, increased demand will be placed on these systems for increased physical fitness; and today evidence supports the theory that increased physical health leads to increased mental health.

*"One of the most often cited benefits of a regular program of physical activity by enthusiastic participants is that they feel better. They report having more energy after exercise, they feel more relaxed and most mention an increased ability to cope with the problems of living. Objective measurements of such psychological changes are difficult to obtain; however, there is no doubt that many participants do temporarily enhance psychological status by engaging in one of a variety of conditioning or vigorous leisure time activities. For many individuals, young and old alike, improvements in*

*physical fitness and appearance by regular exercise yield improvements in self-esteem and self-confidence."*[1]

This book will serve as an excellent reference for professionals treating patients as well as for individuals interested in a personal exercise program and of course for exercise groups and classes. Bob has addressed a chapter especially to teachers of exercise classes.

Although the title addresses only the elderly, clearly these exercises are appropriate as well for younger people who, for any reason, find themselves in a weakened state of health Those recuperating from a period of prolonged bed rest, those who have become weakened due to a

---

[1] William L. Haskell, Ph.D., "Physical Activity in Health Maintenance", Ways of Health, ed. by David Sobel, (New York: Harcourt Brace Jovanovitch, Inc., 1979) p. 454.

chronic debilitating disease, or those recovering from an acute injury will also find the exercises in this book helpful. As complications could arise, I would like to underscore what Bob has pointed out countless times in the book. Your physician should be consulted before undertaking a regular exercise program such as this.

In order to function smoothly, the human body must be exercised. In order to attain and maintain optimum physical and mental health, a regular program of physical exercise is essential. It is our hope that this regular program of physical exercise will be enjoyable for you and that it will help you become the best person you can be.

Marina Brown, RPT

# Preface

After spending most of my adult life exercising on my own and being involved in various levels of professional fitness programs, I was hired to conduct exercise classes in retirement homes and convalescent hospitals. I proceeded to develop my own exercise program under the best of all conditions, right in the facilities with the people. Response has been so positive I decided to put my program in a book.

The exercise program in this book is for older adults, whether they are able to walk or are restricted to a wheelchair or bed and whether OR NOT they have the use of all their limbs. (Actually, the exercises in this book can be used by any age group.) I've re-introduced exercise through my classes to many hundreds of older adults. My oldest student is ninety-nine. One of my classes of twenty people has an average age of seventy-eight. So you see, you're just NOT too old! I'm not about to let you use age as a cop-out.

The basic program is designed so all you need is a straight backed (kitchen) chair. If you're confined to a wheelchair, then you'll be able to perform the exercises while in your wheelchair. There's also a chapter for those confined to a bed. I have also included some exercises using aids which can be made or found right in your own home.

It has been my experience that those who incorporate this program into their lives in a consistent manner feel better physically. They also retain function of usable body areas longer and their morale and social interests improve.

In short, some good, old fashioned fun has returned to their lives. It's my hope that you, too, will soon join them.

R.H.J.

# 1   Getting Started

We all live our lives differently. Because of this and hereditary differences, we are all at various levels of physical condition. There are numerous existing charts which I could have used which provide levels of acceptable weight *vs.* height, pulse *vs.* age *vs.* duration of activity and so on, but these have a tendency to be boring and confusing.

In an effort to keep this program logical and easily understood, charts and graphs have been eliminated. If you need a progress chart you can develop your own by simply recording date, elapsed time and exercises completed, or you can talk to your doctor. I do believe you should, in some way, keep track of your progress. Actually, the most important progress graph you'll need is that look of delight and wonder you'll get from friends and relatives when they see your renewed vim and vigor.

## Where Can I Exercise?

This exercise program has been assembled so that almost anybody can do all or some of it. It was developed so all you need is a kitchen chair and perhaps a broom stick. (No halloween jokes, please.) The program evolved in a classroom format with people in wheelchairs, people with paralyzed limbs and people who were elderly (or just feeling "plain old"). It has been tested and altered to the present form. There is something for everyone in this program. You have no excuse not to begin! Surely you have or can borrow a straight backed chair, broom and space enough to swing your arms around.

## You're Too Old? Too Young?

To put it simply, the purpose of this book is to present an exercise program whereby any person _____ (put your age in the blank) years old can improve his or her physical condition.

The need for exercise knows no age limitations. The program of exercises beginning in Chapter 2 also knows no age limitation. Exercise classes today contain students from ALL AGE GROUPS. I hope that those of you who are younger also recognize your need to exercise regularly. There are many books on the market which provide excellent plans for young and middle aged persons. There are few (I found none) for those of you now in the "Older Adult" group. I'm certain the enclosed program would be beneficial regardless of your age. No, you're not too young and you're certainly not too old.

## Yes, You Have The Time

This exercise program takes approximately forty minutes, (if you do the whole program) three times a week. That's only about .017% of your waking hours so don't tell yourself you haven't got the time. Some of you will find a few of the exercises difficult at first. Don't worry if you are unable to complete the whole program in the beginning. Actually, whatever the number of exercises and the number of times you are able to repeat them will be YOUR beginning. If you are able to do some arm, leg, lung, heart and back exercises for even twenty minutes, you will have established a good base upon which you can build.

The starred (*) exercises provide just such a base to begin with. You should not attempt to get through the whole program "in record time" during your first week. TAKE IT EASY, build up capacity and speed SLOWLY, and concentrate on doing the exercises correctly.

Reasons For Exercising

The purpose of this exercise program is to improve heart and lung condition and capacity, to maintain and improve range of motion (flexibility) and endurance, to avoid muscle and bone weakness (atrophy), decubitus ulcers and constipation. Again, increase your capacity SLOWLY.

This program is designed in such a way that each area of your body is warmed-up before it is subjected to any stress or stretching.

If you are walking but not doing any other exercises, keep on walking and do my program on alternate days or just before going on your walk.

If you are already exercising I'm sure you'll find additional exercises in this book to add to your program. It's essential that your exercise program cover all of your joints, muscles and tendons.

## Getting Started

The enclosed program accompanied by walking, swimming, riding a stationary bicycle or any other similar activity which works your heart will provide the necessary level and range of exercises to keep your body fit from head to toe.

If you are currently in poor condition begin by using just the starred exercises and by walking down to the corner and back. Then in two weeks walk around the block once (approximately a quarter mile). Do this at least three or four times a week.

Build up gradually to additional exercises and longer walks. (If you are unable to walk be certain you do all the leg and feet exercises in the program to the best of your ability.) Build up the length of your walks GRADUALLY over a period of months. Build up the length of your exercise program GRADUALLY over a period of months. Yes, I said MONTHS! TAKE YOUR TIME!

You say you haven't got months? Sure you do. Take some of them to get yourself feeling better. Then keep exercising to **KEEP ON** feeling better.

Discuss this program with your doctor. He'll know whether you should delete or add some exercises because of a personal limitation. He might also suggest (if you bring it up) that you supplement your diet with various vitamins and minerals. Believe me, he'll be happy to help you.

I'm not going to help you exercise or find a chair. I want you to ignore those "helpful" friends and relatives who want you to "take it easy" right into a premature grave. Nobody can help you but yourself; nobody can get you started in a regular exercise program but yourself; nobody can make this vital decision but yourself. I want you to enjoy your body and life. This can happen only when you're mentally and physically active. This process has already begun as you read this book.

I don't want any of you telling yourself you're too old. YOU'RE NOT!

Don't Sleep On It

If you're reading this book YOU HAVE BEGUN. Don't misunderstand me, just reading this book won't help. In fact, sleeping with it under your pillow won't even help. Unless the book disturbs your sleep and you get up and start exercising.

If you have stiff and sore muscles and joints you're going to have to do some consistent work. This means consistent and gradual increase of exercise over a period of time before your stiffness and soreness fades away.

Just like a football player or any other athlete, you're going into "training". Training so you can begin to LIVE again. Training so you can SELL YOUR ROCKING CHAIR.

No Miracles Involved

I am not presenting some magical plan for health and vigor. This book does not contain a secret formula just translated from the scrolls of Tibetan Monks. It does, however, present a way to get the motor of your body tuned up, greased up and running as it was meant to. Note: your friends and relatives may think a miracle has happened. (P.S.: you may share the magical formula contained in this book with them if you wish.)

Certain program limitations may be necessary because of your age or physical problems. These you must take into consideration when deciding what you can realistically expect to accomplish. A trip to your family doctor will help. I assure you he will be happy to learn you've decided to exercise. (Maybe you can convince him he should start exercising, also.)

Doctor's Approval First

If you have high blood pressure, a heart condition, a weight problem, an inoperative limb, arthritis, emphysema or some other medical problem then you must approach this exercise program carefully, with your eyes open and with your doctor's approval.

## Some Medical Considerations

FIRST of all, if you have high blood pressure, a heart, lung or circulatory problem, arthritis or emphysema talk to your doctor and show him this exercise program. He'll tell you which exercises to eliminate, if any, and what other exercises you might possibly add and how many repetitions to perform.

SECOND, if you have a weight problem this will change your approach to the exercises. It is important for you to include some walking. This program is not designed to help you lose weight. However, if you exercise regularly and begin to feel better, perhaps you'll be motivated to do something about the weight. In fact, I know you will. You'll want to look as good as you feel.

THIRD, if you have had a stroke or other injury and part of your body is paralyzed, don't let that stop you from exercising. That's all the more reason to exercise. You've got to maintain, and hopefully, improve what mobility and the level of self-help you currently possess. You should, in fact, even move the paralyzed limb during your exercise period. This will increase the flow of blood and oxygen into the limb. You want to do all you can to keep circulation flowing as freely as possible. You need to exercise to keep your morale up and to maintain a positive mental attitude to fight off natural tendencies of discouragement and depression.

FOURTH, if you are one of those people who have lived into their seventies, eighties or even nineties and think you no longer need to exercise,

THINK AGAIN! Remember, your body is composed of living tissue that needs to be used. If the blood is circulated and the muscles, tendons and joints are activated you will be doing a lot toward fighting off deterioration due to lack of use. Our bodies were built for use, SO USE YOURS.

<u>Is There A Hurry?</u>

The only hurry is beginning. Don't make excuses, START NOW! However, you are urged to begin this exercise program with a realistic attitude. If you have been relatively inactive for a long time then TAKE YOUR TIME. If you're active in some areas, that is, you do your own shopping and cleaning house, etc., then TAKE YOUR TIME. If you walk a little, just for exercise...still TAKE YOUR TIME.

The male model in the exercise photographs walks up to three miles a day, so he, believing he was in top condition, jumped right into this exercise program. Within a few days he had soreness in his lower legs. This was because he was using (exercising) those muscles in a different manner than that provided by walking. He slowed down and the soreness went away in a few days. So TAKE YOUR TIME. Don't be impatient, you'll get there.

Why Take My Time?

Are you beginning to get the hint? This exercise plan will involve some joints, muscles and tendons which your current daily life does not affect. You must, therefore, TAKE YOUR TIME for their sake. If you don't and you hurt some area of your body you might get discouraged and quit. That we don't want! Begin with the starred exercises and take a short walk. If you have any doubts or questions (I repeat!) talk to your doctor.

Take months to work your way up to the full program and a long walk if necessary. You're not competing with anyone except yourself. Follow this plan for the long haul and the result will be an improved use of your body and an improved mental attitude. In other words, you'll enjoy life more.

Exercise With Someone

One tool which you can use is that of exercising with someone else. This provides someone to talk with and someone who can encourage you and vice versa. You could even get a group started in your neighborhood, club or church. (There's more on this in Chapter 7.)

Remember, each of you is on a different level as far as physical condition is concerned so DON'T COMPETE. Just because your neighbor can do a certain exercise ten times doesn't mean you should be able to also. Compete against yourself and the level of activity you could tolerate before you began to exercise. Keep track of your improvement. It's easy to make your own chart.

Now, don't just think about it. Go get a kitchen chair and begin. And remember...TAKE
     YOUR
       TIME

# 2  The Basic Exercise Program

The starred exercises are for new students. You should begin SLOWLY and gradually increase the number of exercises you perform until you can complete the whole program (or as far as you are able). This should take four to eight weeks depending on your physical condition at the time you start the program.

Don't race from one exercise to the other. Take your time. The forty minutes provides adequate time to rest. But not too much!

<u>REMEMBER, if you have a heart condition consult your doctor before doing any exercise which requires you</u>

to move your hands above your head.
*1.
Sit erect on the edge of your chair and place your hands over your lower ribs and upper abdomen. Keep your shoulders down, your elbows straight out and your fingers rigid.

EXHALE while applying firm pressure against your ribs and abdomen with your hands. Exhale slowly through pursed lips (as though you are whistling).

INHALE and expand your chest after releasing the pressure of your hands slightly. Still apply a little pressure against your abdomen. If you have congestion, now is the time to cough gently to raise mucus.

Repeat ten times or as your physician directs.

This exercise is designed to train your abdominal muscles to assist your diaphragm in some of the work of breathing.

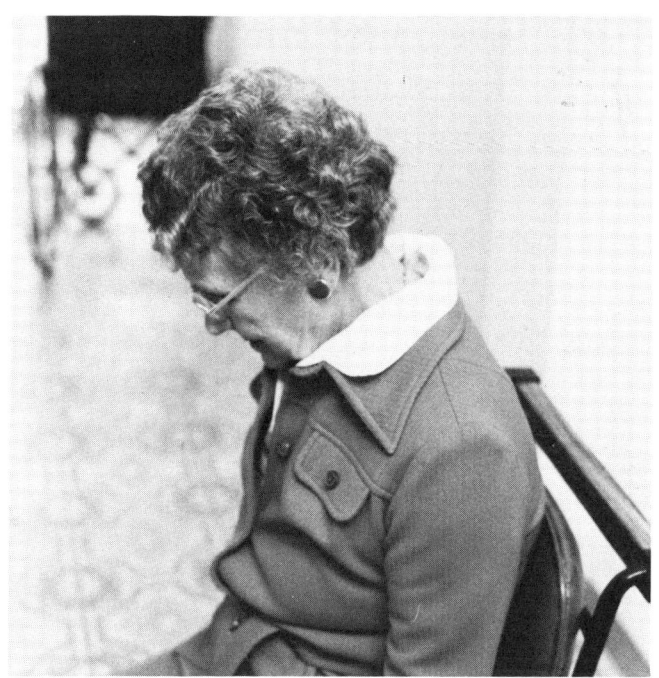

Fig. 1.

\*2

Lower your head toward your chest until it's comfortable. Now move your head to the left and up until it's above your left shoulder; move your head straight across (do not go backwards) until it's above your right shoulder. Move back down to the starting position. Repeat slowly ten times.

Reverse direction of movement and repeat ten times. Do not move your head back behind your shoulders. See Fig. 1.

*3

Move your left ear toward your left shoulder and then your right ear

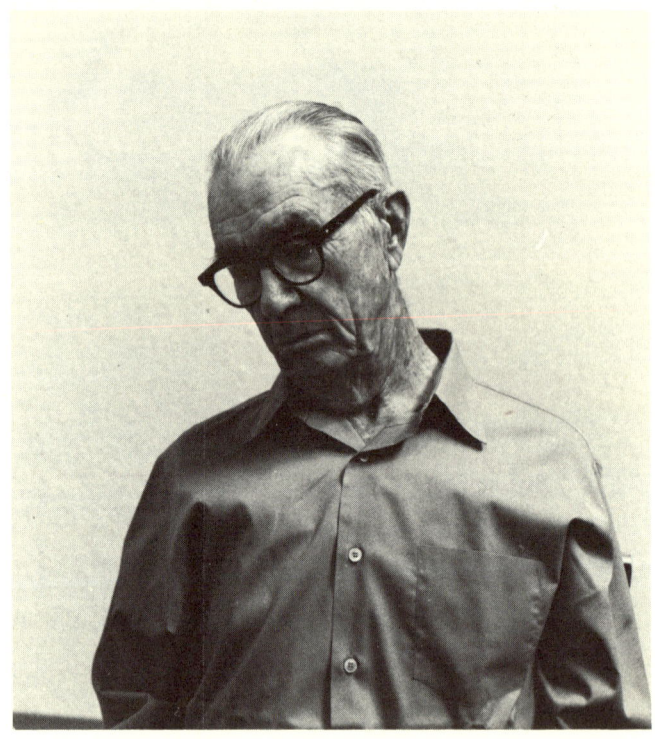

Fig. 2.

toward your right shoulder. Do not move your shoulders.
Repeat ten times to each side.
See Fig. 2.

*4
Move your chin toward your left shoulder and then slowly across and toward your right shoulder. Turn slowly and move as·far left and right as you're able without straining.
Repeat ten times to each shoulder.

*5
Take your right hand and move each finger of your left hand open and closed several times. Now do the same with your right hand.
This will limber the joints of your fingers.
See Fig. 3.

*6
Intertwine your fingers and move your hands left and right. Move them

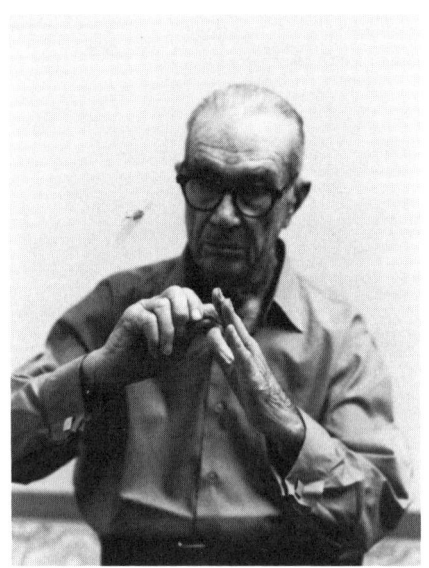

Fig. 3.

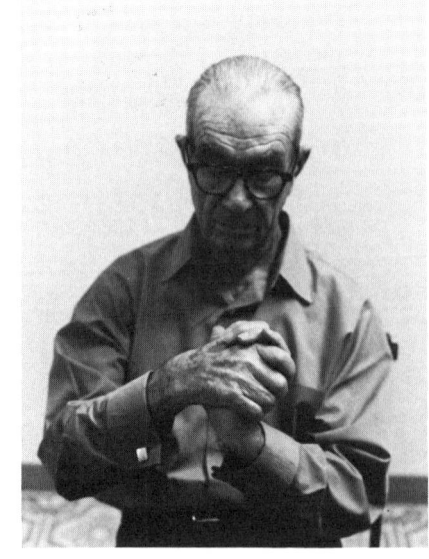

Fig. 4.

in circles to the right and then to the left.
This exercise will limber up your wrist joints. See Fig. 4.

4.
Hold your hands at approximately head or shoulders height. Open your hands and stretch out your fingers as

far as possible. Hold for five seconds. Then make a fist and squeeze it as hard as you can. If you can tighten the muscles of your arms at the same time you will double the benefit.
Repeat cycle three times.
This provides conditioning and limbering for the fingers, hands and arms.
See Fig. 5.

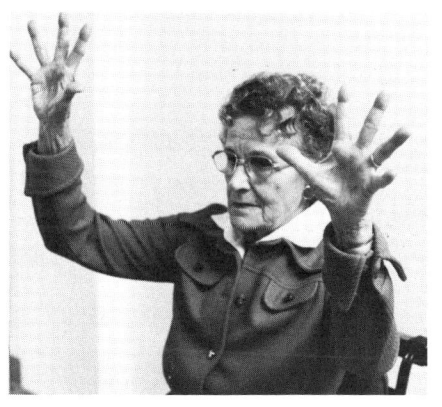

Fig. 5.

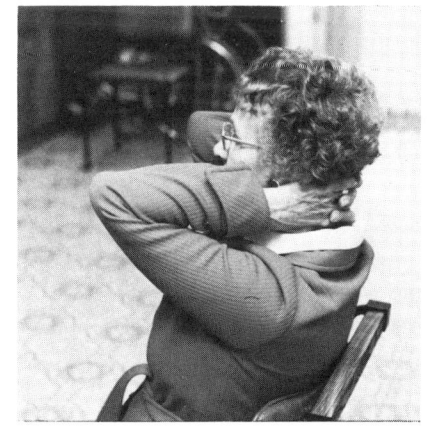

Fig. 6.

7.
Clasp your hands behind your head, keep your hands there while moving your elbows forward and back.
Repeat ten times.
This exercise limbers and conditions upper arm and shoulder joints and muscles.
See Fig. 6. for forward position.

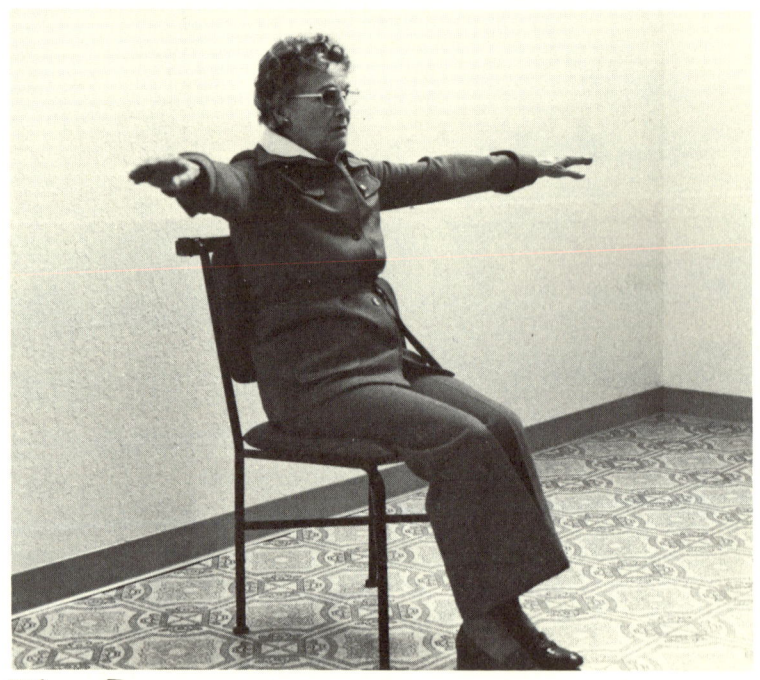

Fig. 7.

\*8
Hold your arms straight out in front, parallel to the floor with your palms together. Now move them straight out to the side keeping them parallel to the floor and then move them back to the front position. Clap your hands as you return them to the starting position. See Figs. 7 and 8.

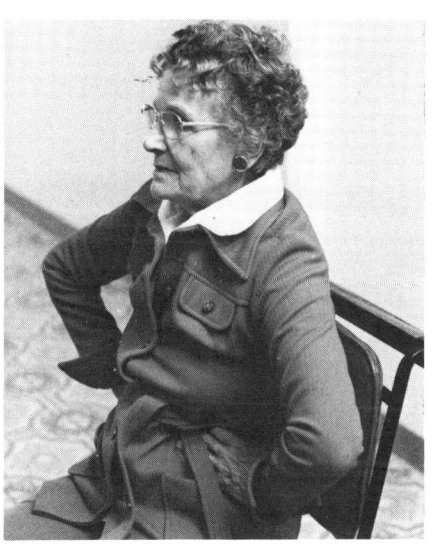

Fig. 9.

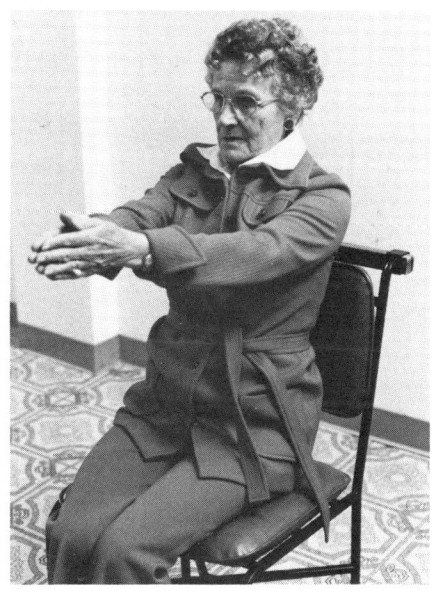

Fig. 8.

*9

Put your hands on your hips. Move your elbows forward and then back.
Repeat ten times.
This stretches upper arm and shoulder muscles.
See Fig. 9. for forward position.

*10.

Relax your arms and let them hang down at your sides. Now gently shake your arms and hands for approximately ten seconds. Now, palms up, raise your hands at least shoulder level. (Raise them above your head with your doctor's approval if you have a heart condition.)
Now lower your arms back to the starting position and start "shaking" again.
Repeat five times.
This exercise promotes circulation in hands and arms (your hands may even tingle). It stretches and

conditions upper arms, trunk and shoulder muscles and joints.
See **Fig. 10** for up position.

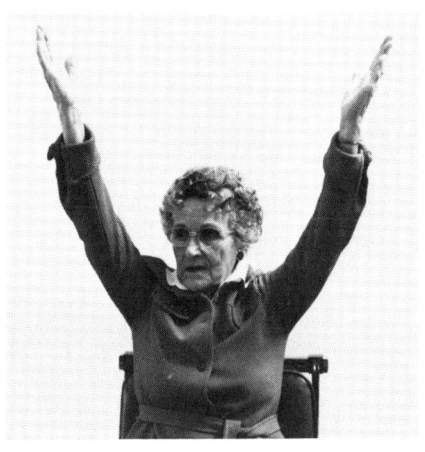

Fig. 10.

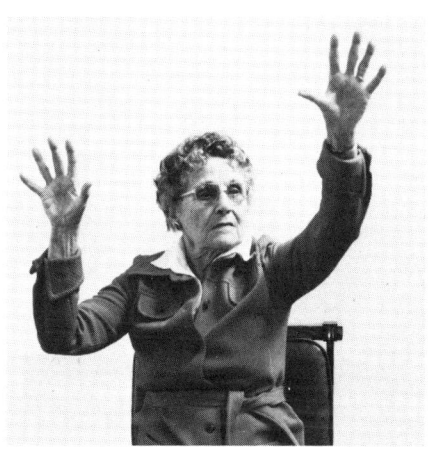

Fig. 11.

11.
Reach up with one arm as high over your head as you're able. Bring this arm down and raise the other arm over your head.
Reach up with each arm ten times.
Be sure to consult your doctor before

doing this exercise if you have a heart condition.

This exercise is used to keep you in condition in case you ever find yourself standing beneath a money tree. This way you'll be able to pick a lot of the "fruit" before becoming tired.

This exercise stretches arm, upper side and shoulder muscles and joints. See Fig. 11.

12.
Reach out in front of you, as though swimming, first with one arm and then the other.

Reach out with each arm ten times. If only one of your arms is able to do this exercise then do it with one arm.

This exercise stretches arm, shoulder and upper back muscles.

See Fig. 12.

13.
Totally relax your left arm. Put your

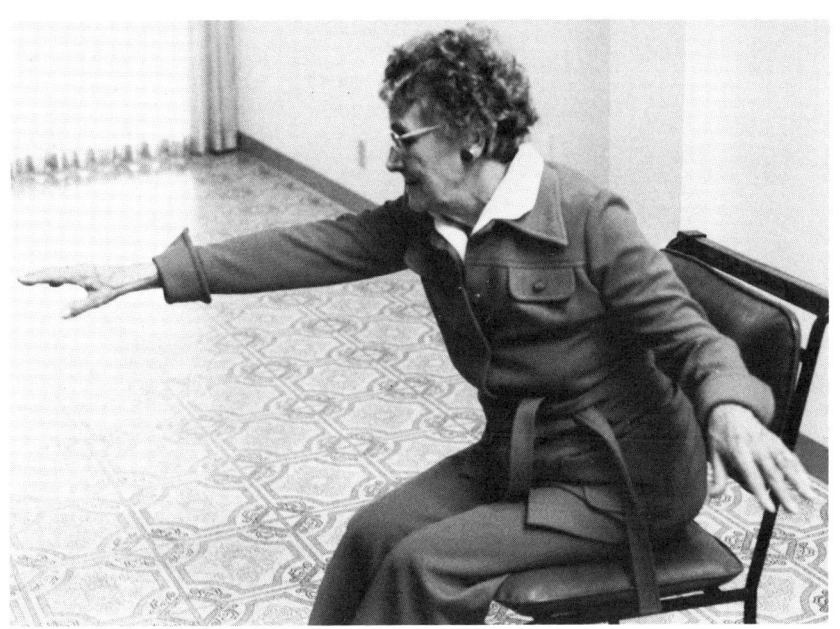

Fig. 12.

right hand under your left elbow and lift the relaxed left arm. Let your right arm do all the work.
Repeat ten times and reverse.
This exercise conditions upper arm muscles.
See Fig. 13. for up position.
*14.
Take your right fist in your left hand. Push the arm straight back along your

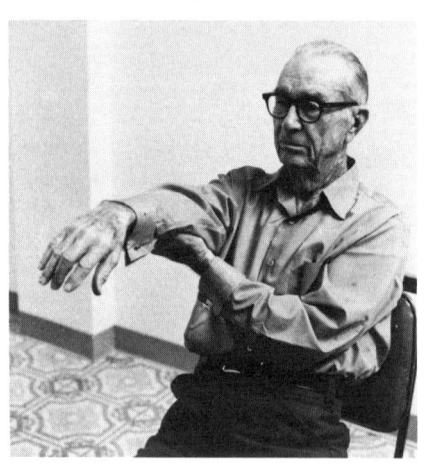

Fig. 13.

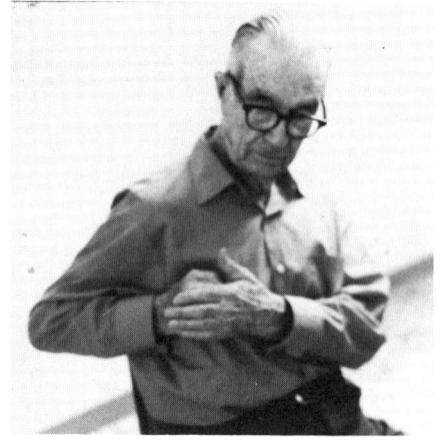

Fig. 14.

right side. Move hands forward and push back again. When moving your hands back to the starting position you can exert a little (or a lot of) pressure against your hands, thereby providing additional conditioning for your arms.

Repeat ten times for each arm.

This exercise provides stretching and conditioning for the whole arm if you

exert pressure when returning to the starting position.
See Fig. 14. for back position.
*15.
Lower your head and let your arms hang at your sides. See Fig. 15.

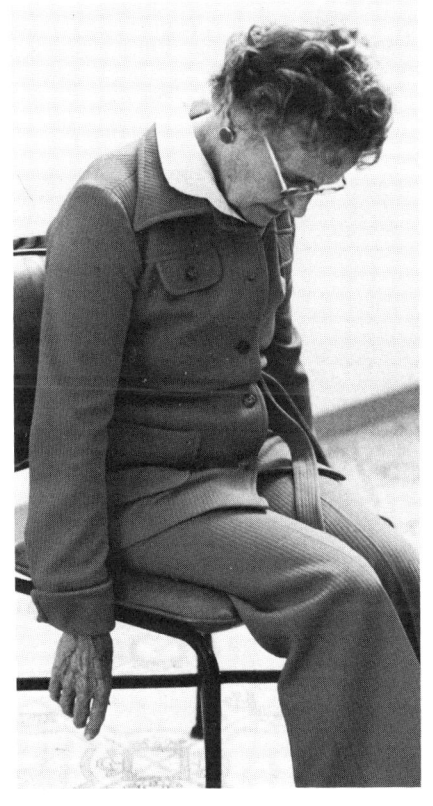
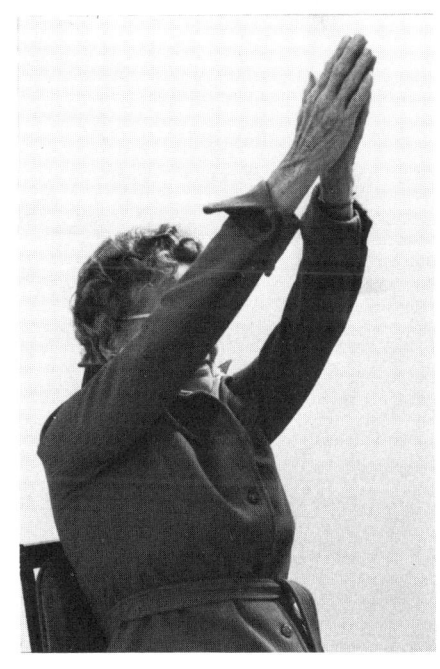

Fig. 15.  Fig. 16.

SLOWLY inhale DEEPLY as you SLOWLY raise your head (do not let your head go back behind your shoulders) and hands above your head. Now, SLOWLY and COM— PLETELY exhale as you lower your head and hands. Repeat four times. This exercise expands and conditions your lungs, and it limbers your arms and neck muscles and joints.

*16.
Put your hands together, lock your elbows (if you can) and put your hands just above your knees. Now raise and lower your arms keeping your hands together and your elbows locked. Keep hands below head if you have a heart condition. Repeat ten times.

This conditions and stretches upper arm, back and shoulder muscles.
See Fig. 16. for upper position.

*17.

Rock-a-by-baby.. Grasp both elbows (or as close as you can come) with both hands and move your arms left and right, moving your elbows out to the side as far as possible. Sing the song and do the exercise at the same time. If you can't sing then hum or whistle.

If you don't know the song, repeat exercise ten times to each side.

See Fig. 17.

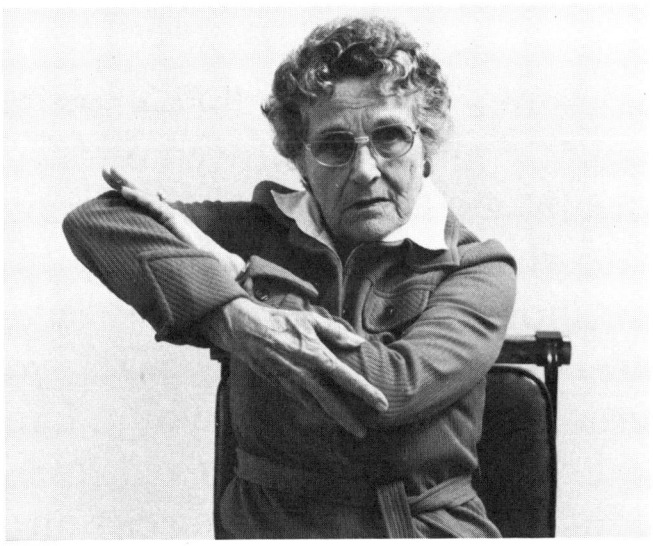

Fig. 17.

*18.
Sit up straight in your chair. Put your hands in your lap and move your shoulders forward, up, back and down. (Sort of a circular movement.) Repeat this circle ten times. Change the direction of the circle and move your shoulders back, up, forward and return to the starting position. Repeat this circle ten times.

This exercise limbers tendons, muscles and joints in your shoulders.

19.
Hold your arms, with elbows straight, down at your sides. Move your arms, with elbows locked, up and straight out to the side. Move them up to at least shoulder height. If you have a heart condition, check with your doctor before raising your hands above your head. Repeat ten times.

This exercise works the muscles on the outside of your shoulders. See Fig. 18.

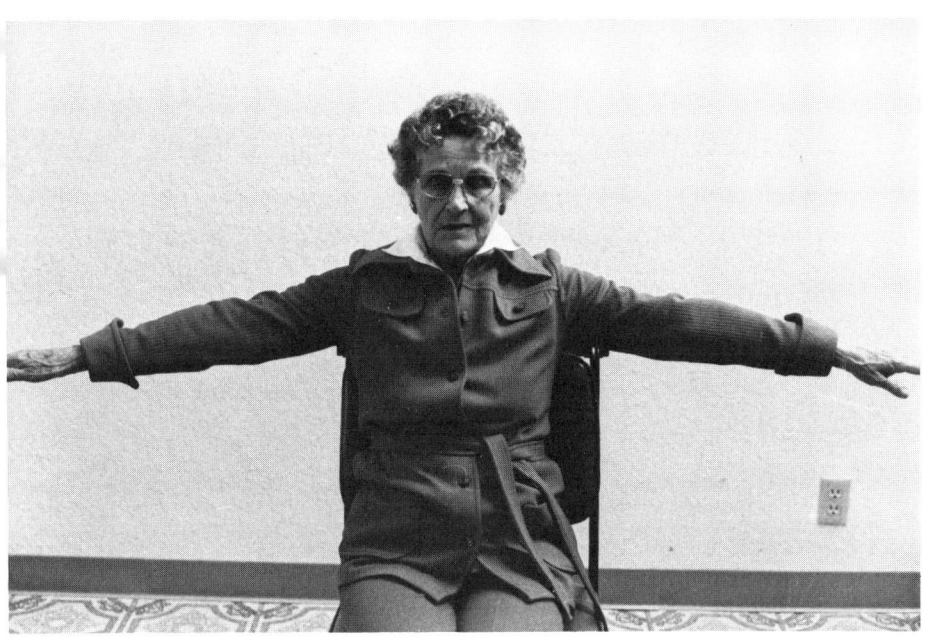

Fig. 18.

*20.

Put your hands on your hips, keep your bottom flat on the chair and lean left and then lean right. Do not lean very far until you've done at least ten repetitions. And, also, if you lean too far you'll end up right in the middle of another exercise...picking yourself up off the floor.

It's very important to begin SLOWLY and warm up.

After those ten warm-up repetitions do five more, increasing the distance you lean a little each time.

This exercise stretches side and back muscles and joints.

See Fig. 19.

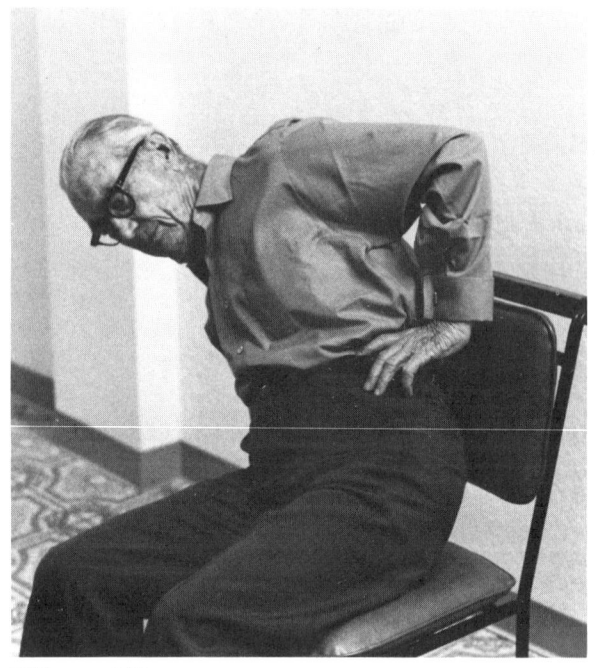

Fig. 19.

*21.
Put your hands on your hips, lean forward and then back to an upright position. Do not lean very far until you've done at least ten repetitions. Again, WARM UP and move SLOWLY at first. Then, after ten cycles, do five more, increasing the distance you lean a little each time. This exercise stretches lower back muscles and joints.
See Fig. 20.

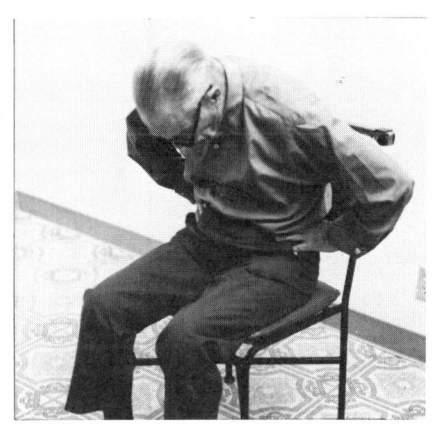

Fig. 20.

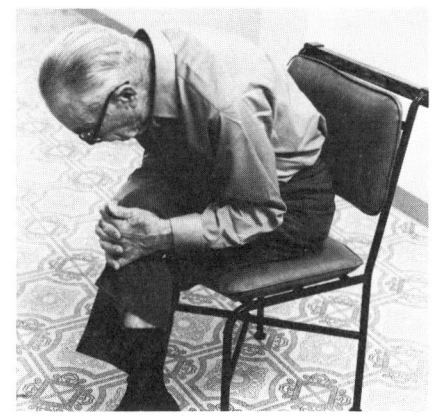

Fig. 21.

22.
Cross one leg over the other knee. Clasp your hands across the front of your upper knee. Now lean forward a little being careful not to lean too far or go too fast. Lean forward at least ten times, warming up, before moving further forward. Now, lean further forward, a little each time, for at least five more times. Remember to move SLOWLY.
Reverse your legs and repeat.
See Fig. 21.
23.
Clasp your hands behind your head. Now SLOWLY lean and stretch to the left and then across to the right.
Repeat ten times to each side.
This exercise stretches and conditions sides, lower back and shoulders.
See Fig. 22.

NOTE:
Remember, if there's ever ANY doubt

about any of these exercises, talk to your doctor.
24.
Put your hands on your hips. Twist your body to the right side and then to the left. When you twist, move your arms and head as well. If you've done the previous exercises, you're warmed up and will enjoy this one.
Repeat ten times to each side.
This exercise will stretch and limber up your trunk.
See Fig. 23.

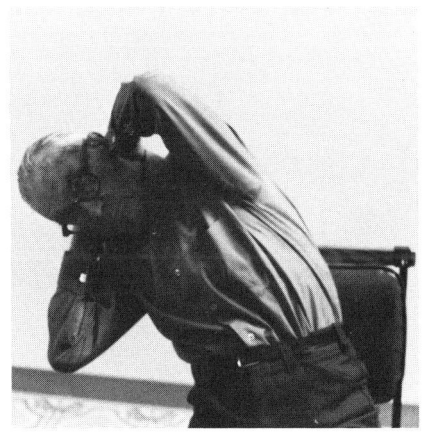

Fig. 22.

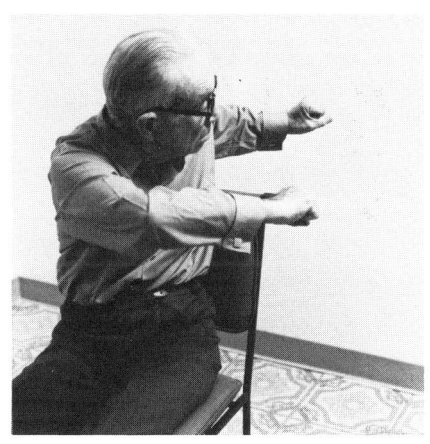

Fig. 23.

25.
Clasp your hands behind your head, bend over and stretch your elbows toward your knees, then sit up SLOWLY. Repeat ten times.

If there's ANY doubt, get permission from your doctor before attempting this exercise.

This exercise stretches and conditions back muscles and joints.

See Fig. 24.

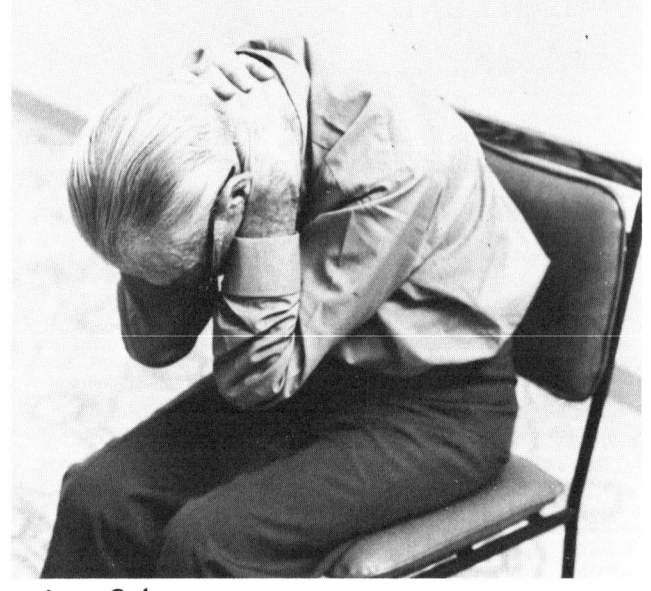

Fig. 24.

*26.

Sit still and bounce your feet on the floor, touching first one foot and then the other. Move them (or one leg if the other is paralyzed) up and down as fast, hard and long as you wish or are able. Do not, however, allow yourself to become over-tired. There's still a lot of exercises to do.

This gets the blood and oxygen flowing through your legs into your feet.

*27.

Sit with your feet flat on the floor. First, raise your heels off the floor while keeping your toes down.

Repeat twenty times.

Second, raise your heels off the floor but keep your toes down and then raise your toes off the floor keeping your heels on the floor. This creates a kind of rocking movement. If there's enough of you in the class you can get

a nice rhythm going if you all do it together.
Repeat twenty times.
See Fig. 25. for heels up position.

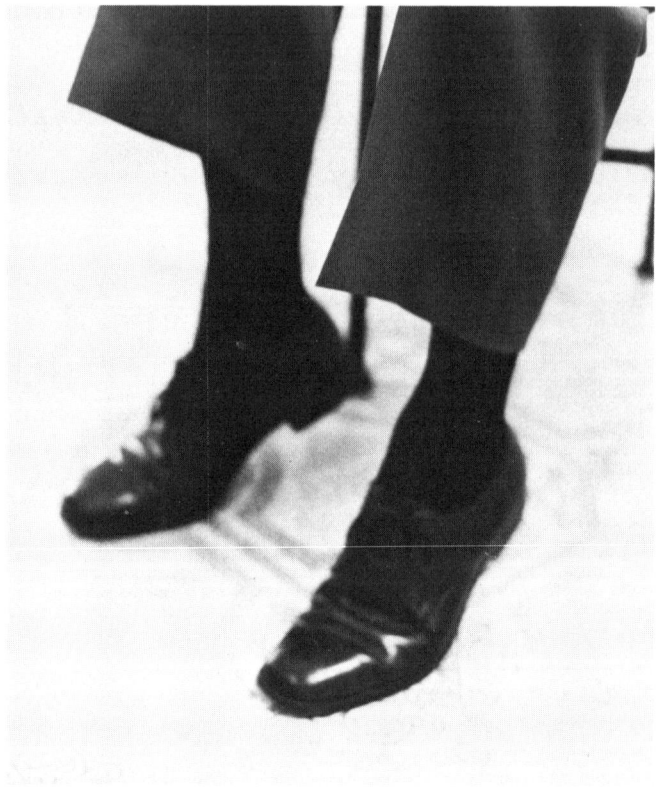

Fig. 25.

28.
Hold your legs off the floor and straight out in front. Straighten your knees if you can.
See Fig. 26.

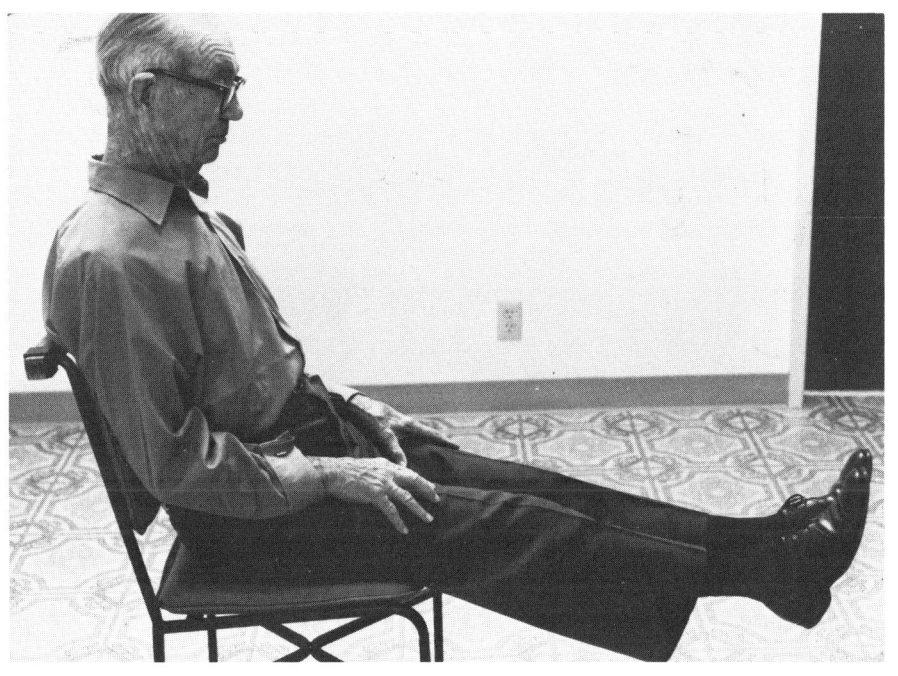

Fig. 26.

Now, point your toes out away from you like a dancer. Move your feet up and down in a walking movement See Fig. 27.

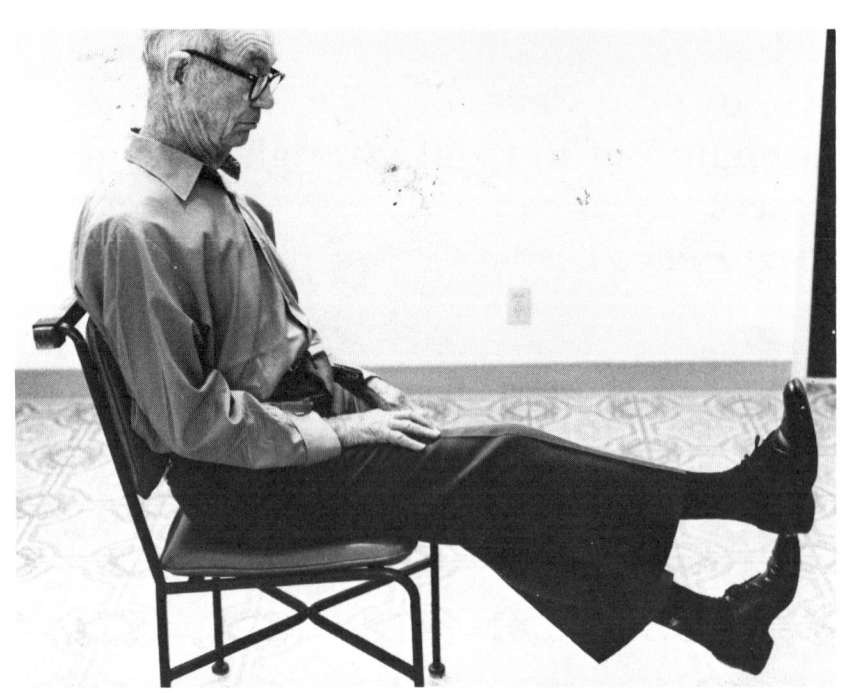

Fig. 27.

Move each leg up and down ten times. You can add more repetitions to this exercise as your physical condition improves.

This exercise conditions thighs, ankles, lower back and stomach muscles.

*29.

Raise one thigh off the chair as high as

you can and then put it back down on the chair.
Repeat this exercise fifteen times.
Do the same thing with your other leg.
If you are unable to lift one of your

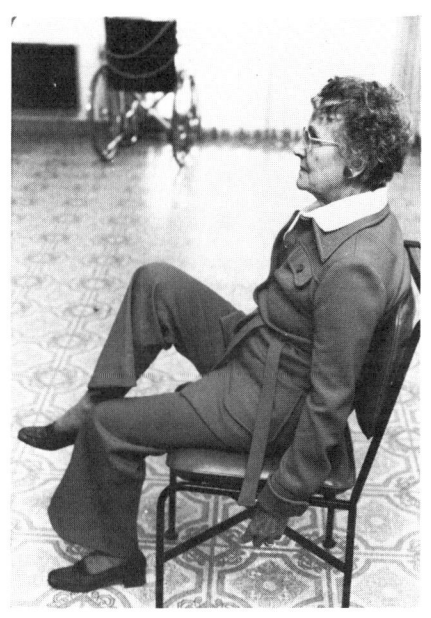

Fig. 28.

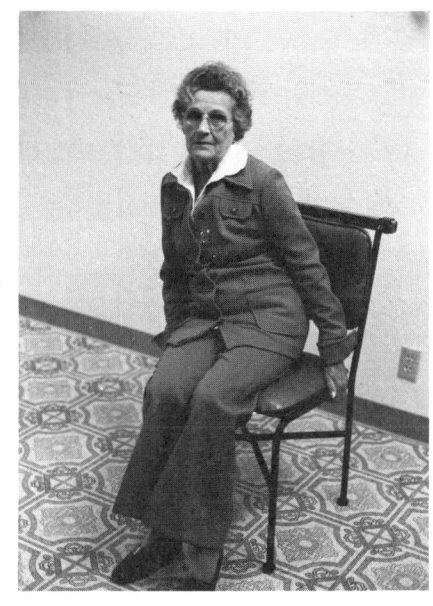

Fig. 29.

legs, use your arms to lift it up and down. The movement will result in increased circulation which will be good for this weakened leg.

This exercise conditions thighs, lower back and stomach muscles.

See Fig. 28.

29-A

This is for those of you who do not walk very much, if at all. Move to your left pushing up with your right leg. This is done to lift the right side of your bottom (or your "sit upon it" as one English lady called it) off your chair. Hold for five seconds. Reverse and lift left side.

See Fig. 29.

30.

Extend one leg and rotate it ten times in one direction and then ten times in the other direction. Try to hold your toes back while circling.

Repeat with the other leg.

This conditions legs, thighs, lower back and stomach muscles.
See Fig. 30.

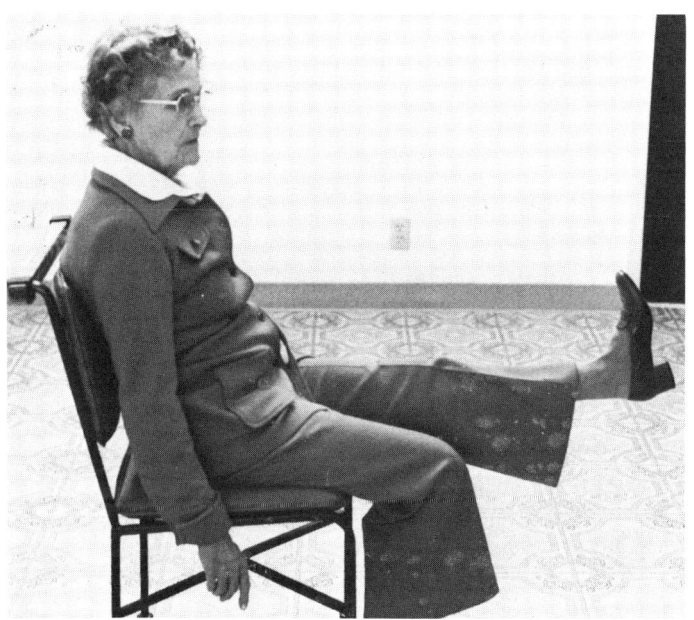

Fig. 30.

31.
Cross your legs at the ankles. Totally relax the top leg and lift it with the bottom leg.
Repeat ten times.
Reverse your legs and repeat ten times.

This exercise conditions thigh, stomach and lower back.
See Fig. 31.

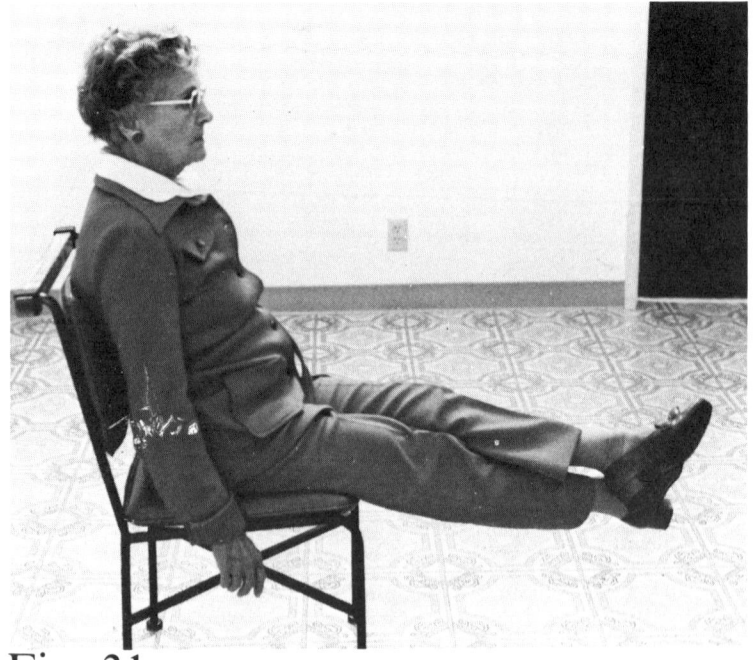

Fig. 31.
32.
Hold your legs straight out in front of you and off the floor. Separate your legs and then move them in a scissoring motion, first right over left and then left over right.
Repeat ten times.

This exercise stretches and conditions upper legs, lower back and stomach muscles.
See Fig. 32.

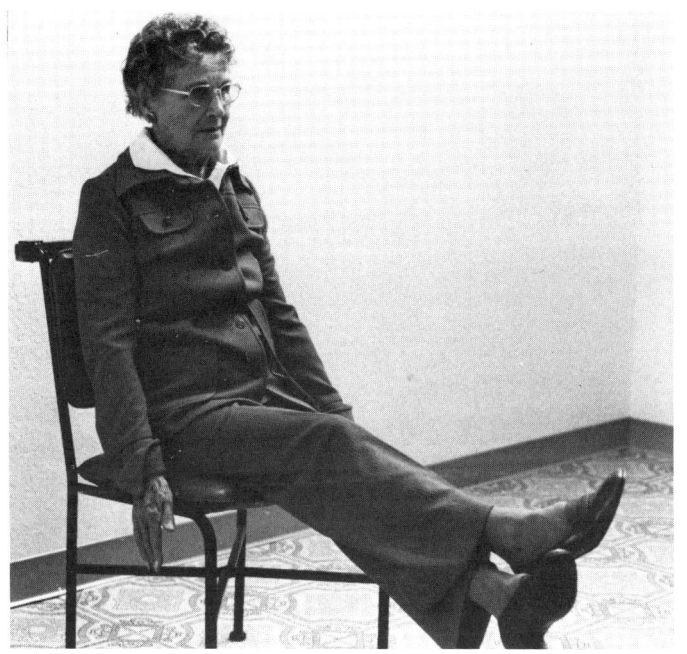

Fig. 32.
33.
Hold your arms straight out to your sides. Circle your arms five times in one direction.
Now raise your legs and "start walking" while you circle your arms

five times in the opposite direction. This exercise, although strenuous, is brief and mainly for co-ordination. See Fig. 33.

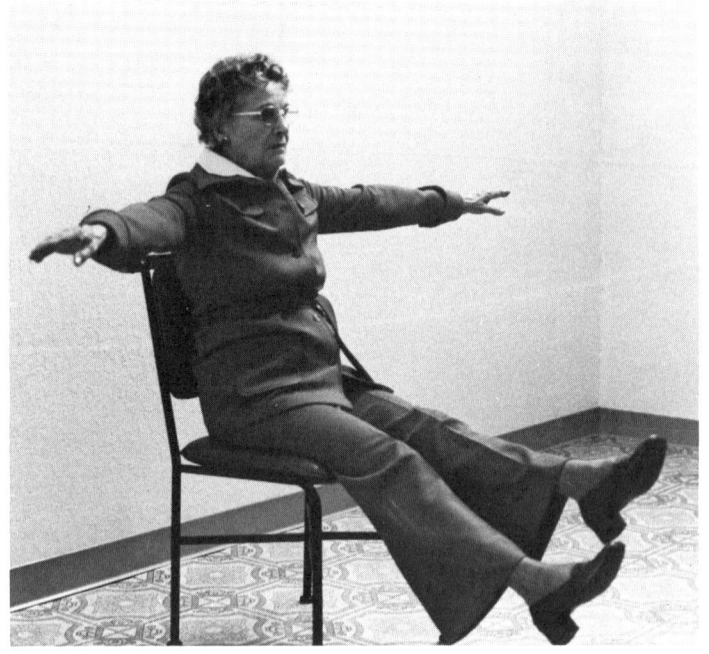

Fig. 33.

*34

One exercise which is very important concentrates on eye-hand co-ordination. I recommend a seven inch in diameter "nerf" (sponge) type ball.

These very soft balls will bounce but will not hurt even in one hits you in the face.

If you're by yourself, sit about three to six feet from a wall but facing it. Throw the ball against the wall and "watch it into your hands". In other words, catch it!
See Fig. 34.

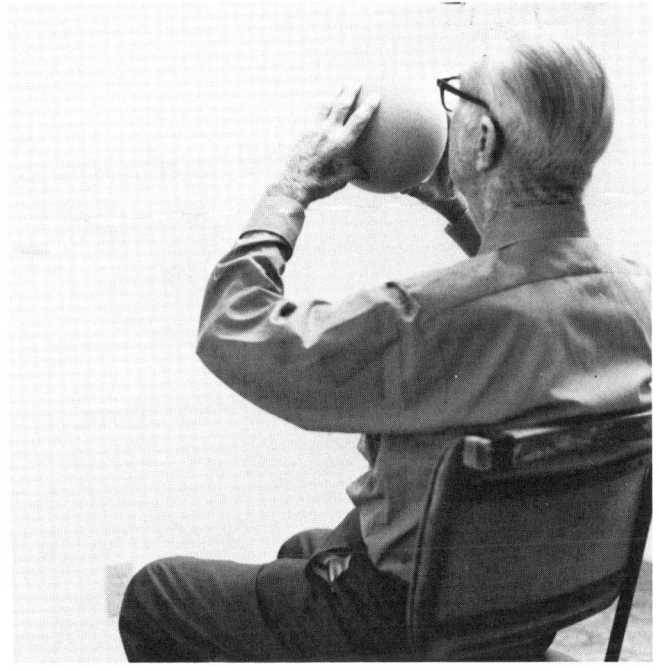

Fig. 34.

If you're with others, sit three to six feet apart and throw the ball back and forth.
See Fig. 34A.

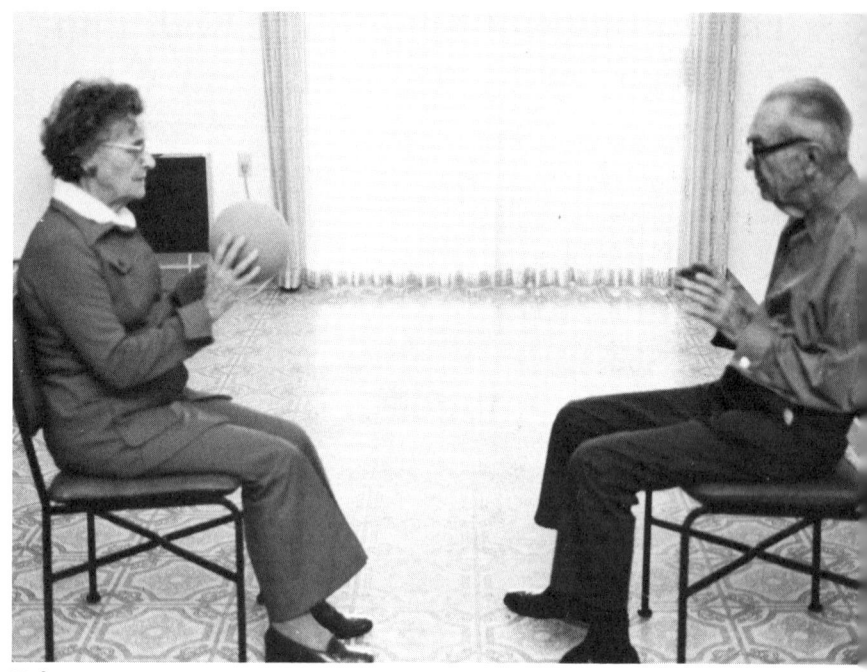

Fig. 34A.

If one of you (or a student) has a paralyzed or missing arm, throw the ball against the wall so it returns to your chest. Bring your other arm up behind the ball there-by catching the ball between your chest and hand.

At this point you should have some questions. Why are there so many leg and feet exercises and why do you stress moving SLOWLY so often?

Help Blood Circulate

There are so many leg and feet exercises because our heart does not, unaided, adequately circulate blood through our legs and feet. Our legs and feet, therefore, require exercise before blood is adequately circulated.

Most of you probably do not jog or play tennis, etc., therefore, my exercise program calls for a considerable amount of time spent stretching and conditioning and thereby helping your heart in the important job of circulating blood through your body.

## Don't Surprise Your Body

By taking your time and moving SLOWLY your muscles, tendons and joints have time to adjust to movement and will, in that way, avoid injury.

If you think enough about your health to make this exercise program part of your life, then you should also think enough of your health to inform your physician and make sure you have permission to do all or most of the exercises described.

I have made no effort in this program to avoid exercises which might tax your current level of condition no matter how good it might be. In fact, I've done just the opposite. I've found most people can do more than they realize. Now, **HAPPY HEALTH TO YOU!**

# 3 A Few Wheelchair Exercises (with aids)

I've included just a few exercises for those of you who have a weakened or paralyzed limb and need special exercises or tools to aid in exercising that limb.

There are two exercise tools that will be helpful in these exercises. The first tool is pictured over the page.

This aid consists of twenty inches of ⅜" o.d. (outer diameter) vinyl surgical tubing with the ends tied together, a ¾" × 6" piece of dowel stick with a ³/₁₆" hole in the middle and a piece of nylon cord to tie the tubing and dowel together. The Figure shows how these items look when put together.

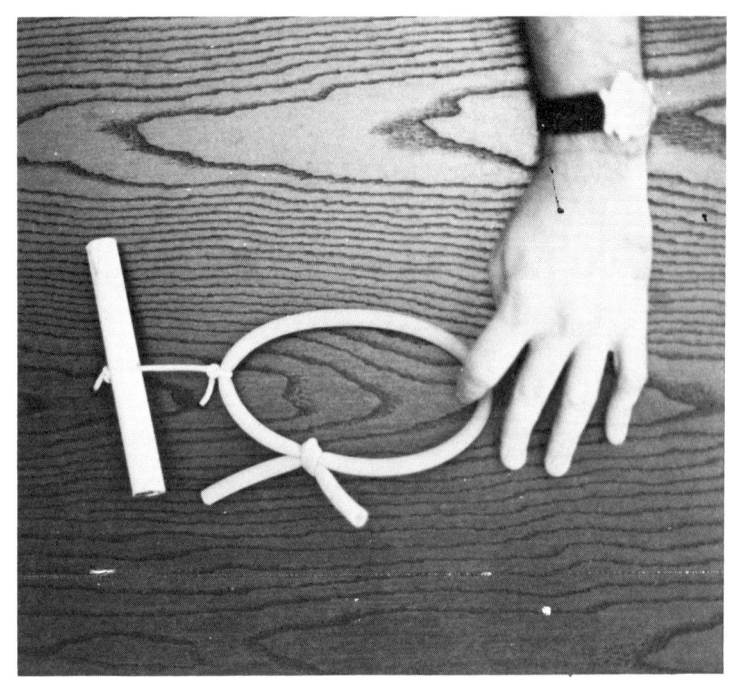

The other exercise tool consists of seven to ten feet of ½" o.d. (or wider) vinyl surgical tubing. Length to be determined by the person's size and the exercises involved. Tie the ends together.

The price for the tool shown above is approximately $2.50. The price for the length of ½" tubing is approximately $6.00. Surgical tubing can be

found at most medical supply stores. So you see, both tools are within most people's budget.
REMEMBER, GO SLOW ON ALL OF THESE EXERCISES.
35.
Loop the short tubing around the wheelchair handle, put the handle

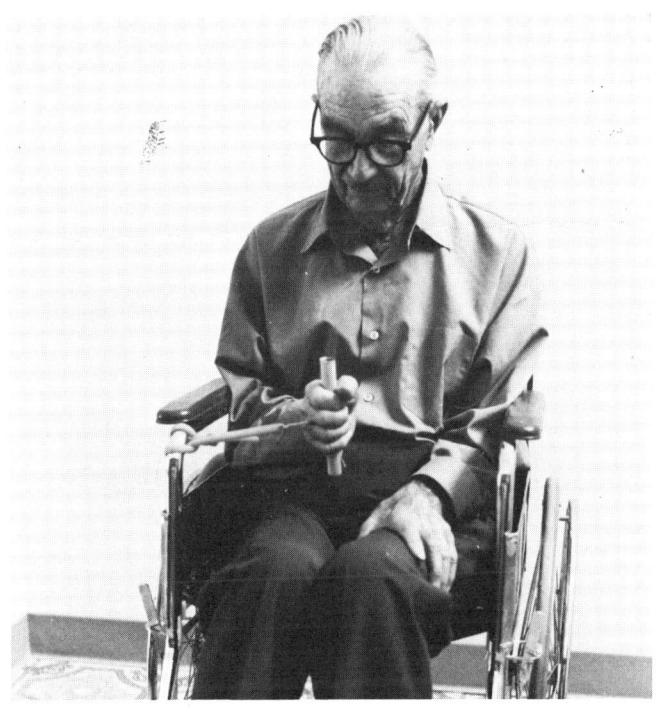

Fig. 35.

through the tubing and tighten. Take the tool's handle in your hand and pull.

Pull ten times, three times a day. Pull only an inch or two at first until your arm's muscles "wake up". Take your time (months if necessary) in building up your arm. It's of the utmost importance that you move slowly. If you don't, you could hurt a muscle or tendon. Then you might quit and that's the last thing I want you to do. Do both arms. SO GO VERY SLOW. See Fig. 35.

36.

Loop the long tubing around one of your wheelchair's push handles, across the back of the chair, under the opposite push handle to your hand. Now pull forward. SLOWLY increase the distance you stretch the tubing. Repeat ten times. Reverse tubing and repeat with other arm.

See Fig. 36.

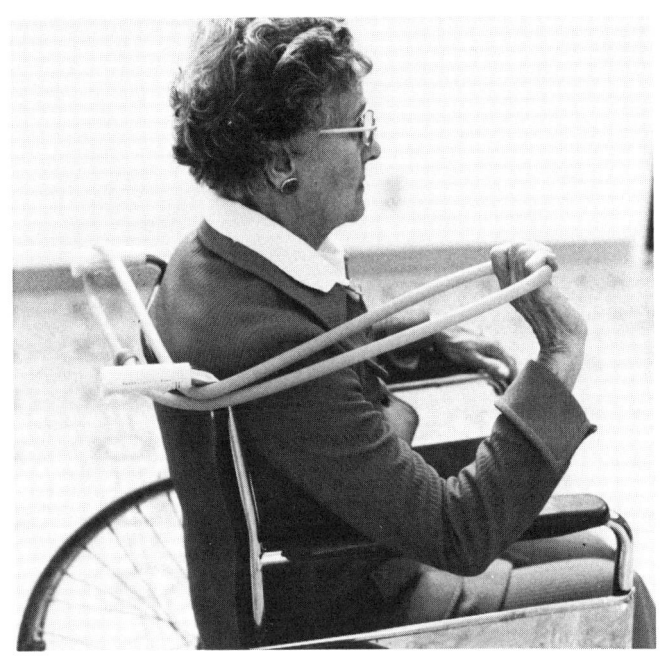

Fig. 36.

37.
Loop the long tubing around one foot pedal of your wheelchair, under the other foot pedal and up to your hand. Now pull up. SLOWLY increase the distance you- stretch the tubing. Increase as the strength of your arm increases. Repeat ten times. Reverse tubing and repeat with other arm. See Fig. 37.

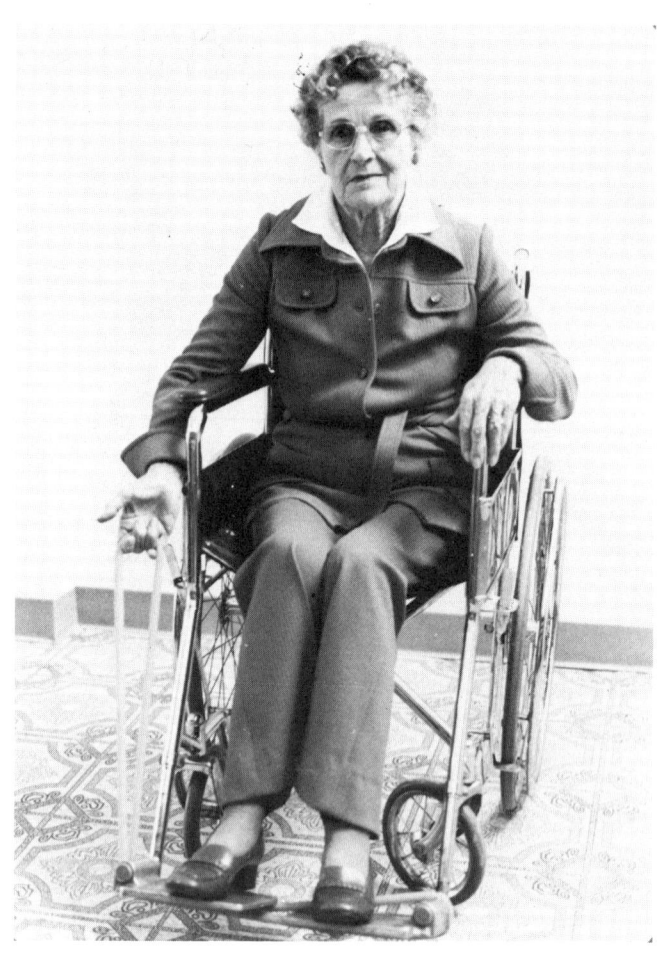

Fig. 37.

38.
Loop the long tubing around one of your wheelchair's push handles and then loop the tubing around one foot.

Now move your foot toward the midline of your body and then away. Reverse and do with other leg. Remember to move slowly.
See Fig. 38. for out position.

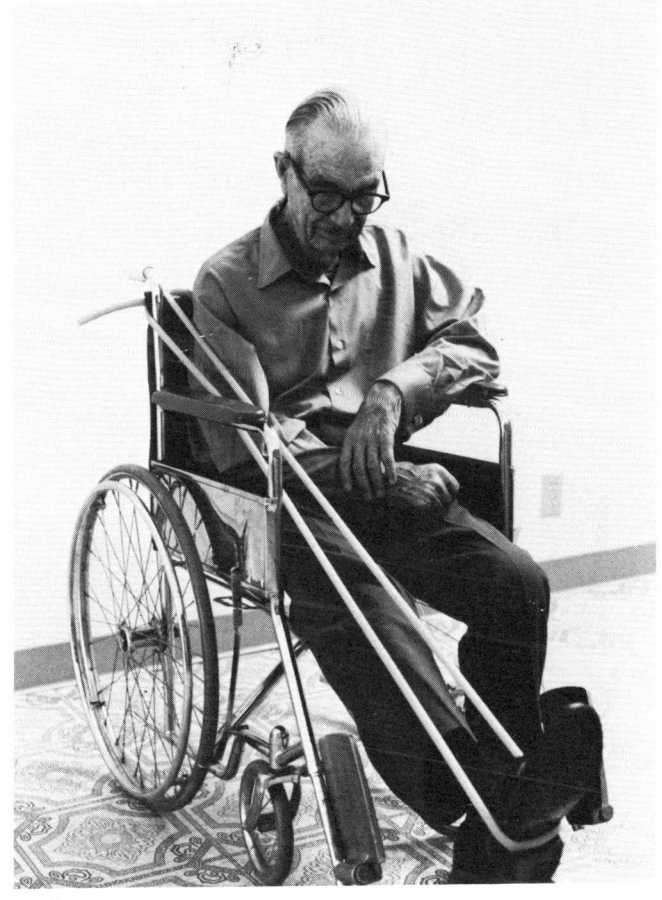

Fig. 38.

I encourage you to have someone with you when you are doing these exercises. They can help you arrange the tubing before each exercise. (This person is NOT to do the exercises for you. That's CHEATING.)

If your ability to help yourself is limited, don't get discouraged. When you start exercising, you should be able to maintain, and hopefully increase, your overall health and your level of self help will improve. Right? RIGHT!

# 4 Exercise Tools and Special Exercises

This chapter provides some additional exercises using our big rubber loop, the small loop tied to the round stick and a three foot long piece of dowel or broom stick. There are also a few exercises for a paralyzed arm or weakened hand and some exercises requiring proper reflexes and response.

<u>Some Stick Exercises</u>
39.
Hold one end of a three foot long, round stick and strike toward the floor while yelling "I don't want to". Hitting the floor isn't necessary. (This

exercise is for classroom use.) Repeat as often as wished.

The purpose of this exercise is to relieve tension for those of you (I need it, too) who feel ready to "burst". See Fig. 39.

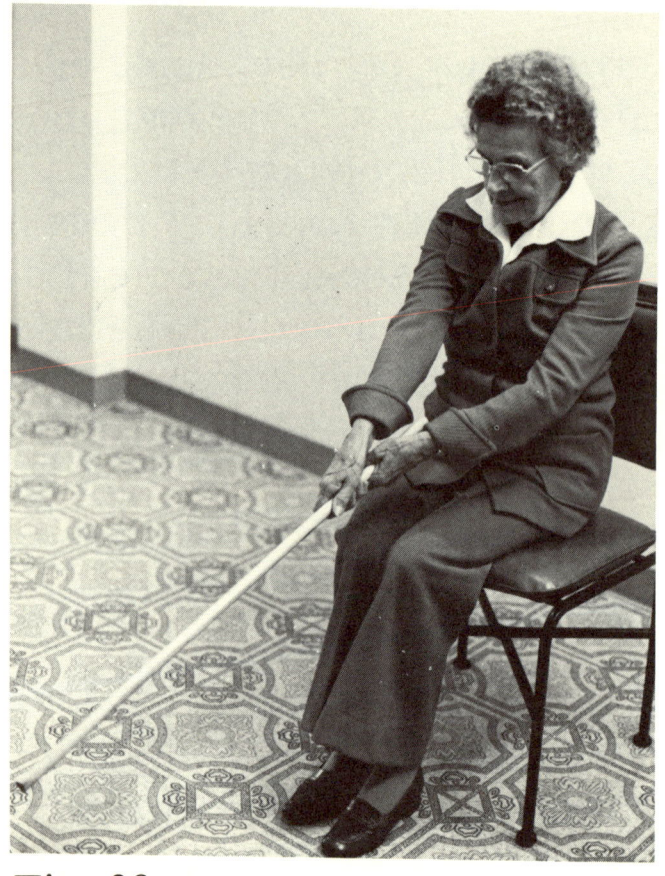

Fig. 39.

40.
Hold each end of the stick in a hand. Now hold the stick over your head and bend left and then right.
Repeat ten times in each direction.

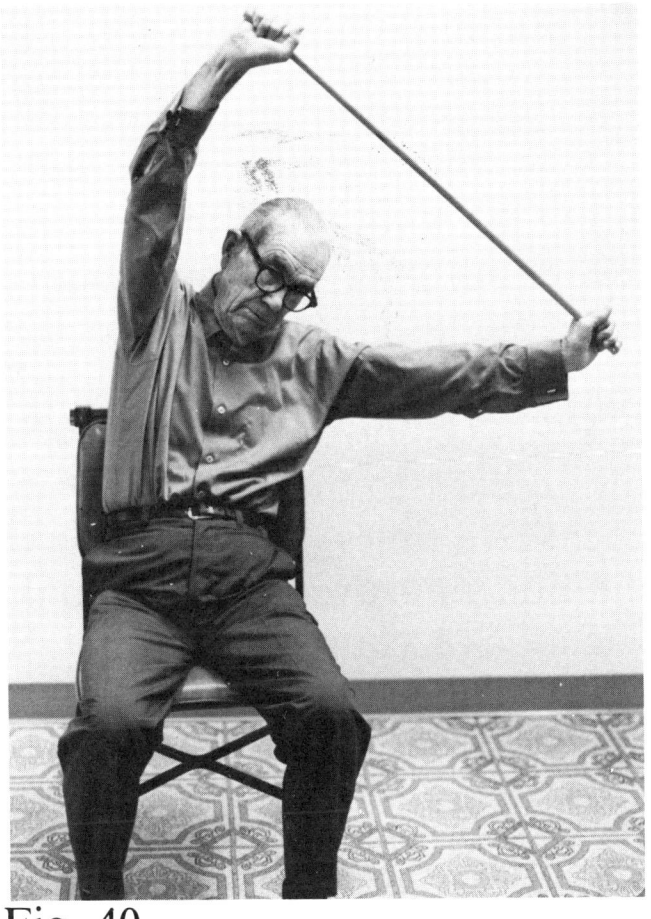

Fig. 40.

This exercise stretches side muscles and tendons and conditions and strengthens arms.

This is a good one to check with your doctor first.

See Fig. 40.

41.

Hold each end of the stick in a hand. Hold the stick up over your head. See Fig. 41A for starting position.

Now bend over moving the stick toward and as close to your ankles as you can.

See Fig. 41B for down position.

Now go back to the starting position. Repeat five times. Add more as your condition improves. This exercise is difficult. See your doctor if you have any doubts about doing it.

This exercise stretches and conditions back and arm muscles.

Some Long Loop Exercises

Grasp the long loop at opposite sides

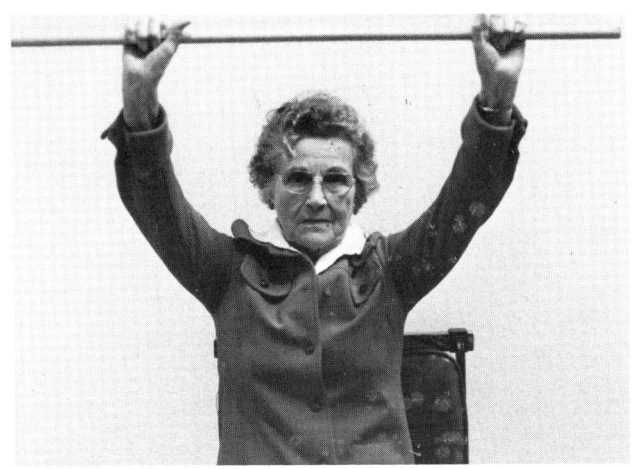

Fig. 41-A.

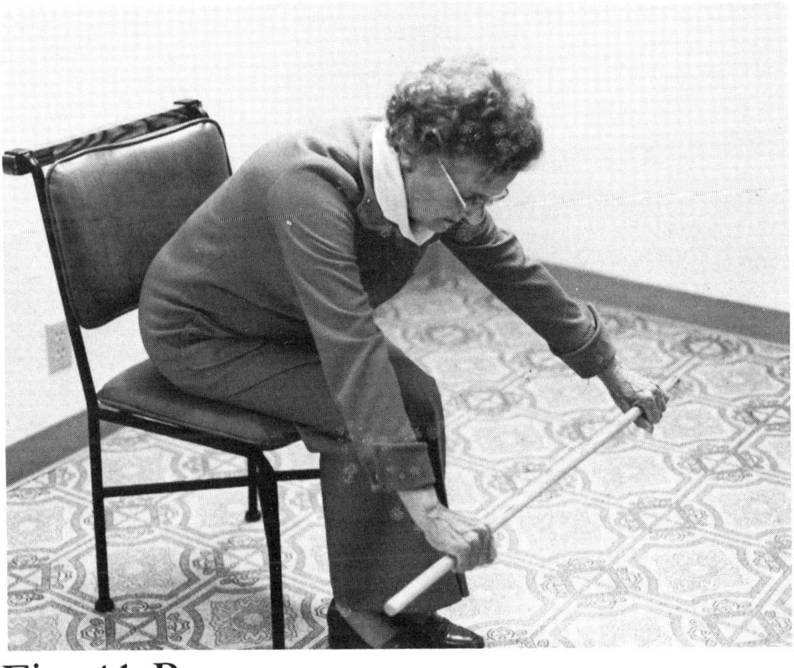

Fig. 41-B.

with both hands. Put the tubing behind your head and SLOWLY pull out to the sides. Now relax the tension and repeat.
Repeat ten times.
See Fig. 42.
43.
Grasp long loop at opposite sides with

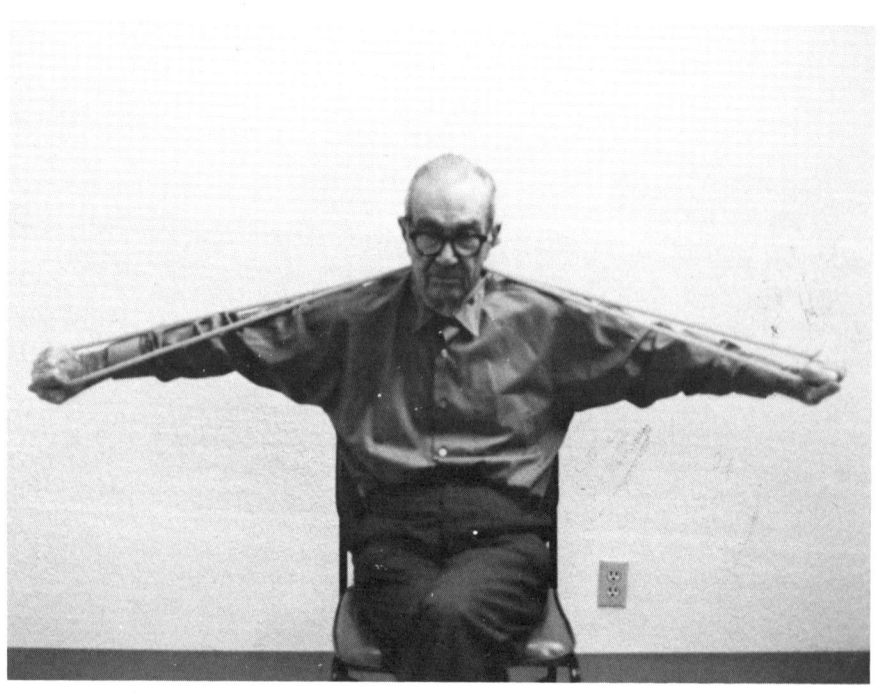

Fig. 42.

both hands in front of your chest. Now pull SLOWLY out to the sides. Relax tension and repeat. Shorten loop as you strengthen.
Repeat ten times.
See Fig. 43.
44.
Put the tubing under both feet. Grasp tubing with palms up and hands about

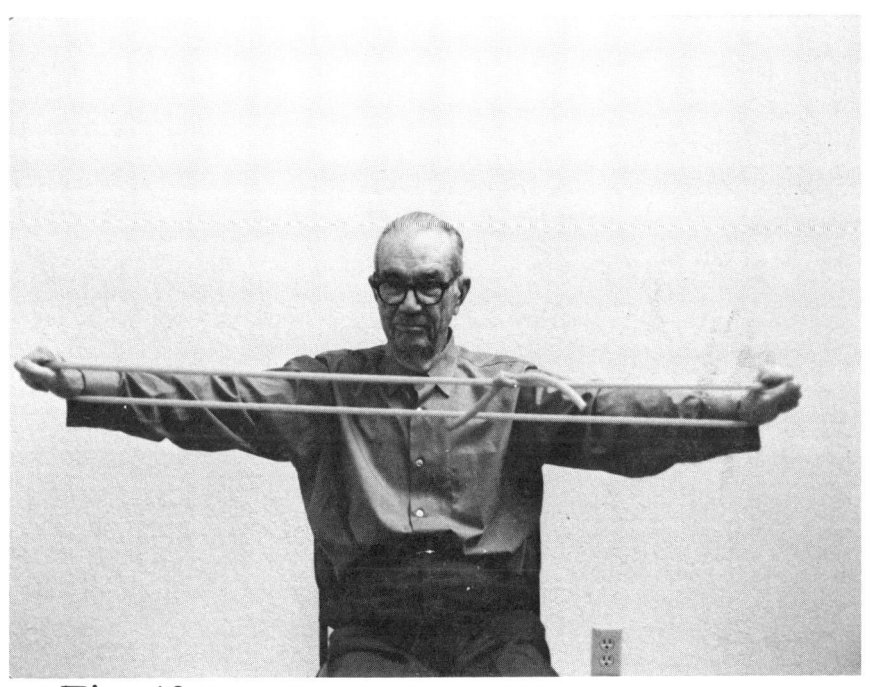
Fig. 43.

six inches apart. Now pull up as far as you can without too much strain. As you become stronger, increase the distance you pull the tubing up. Repeat ten times.
See Fig. 44.

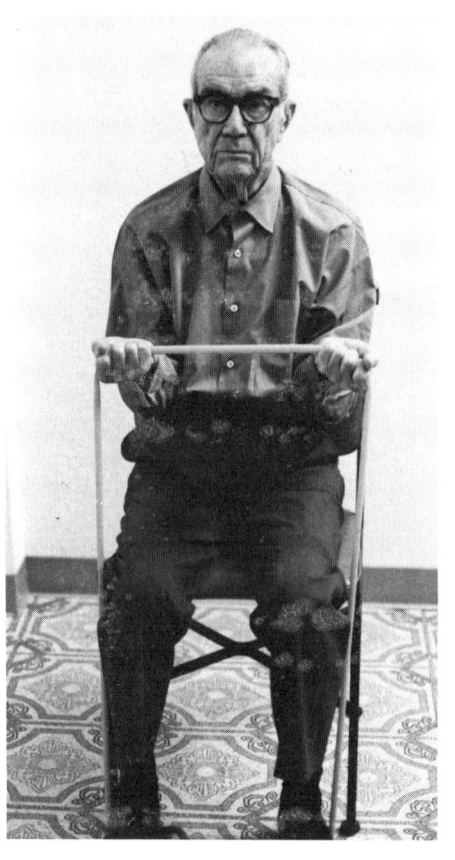

Fig. 44.

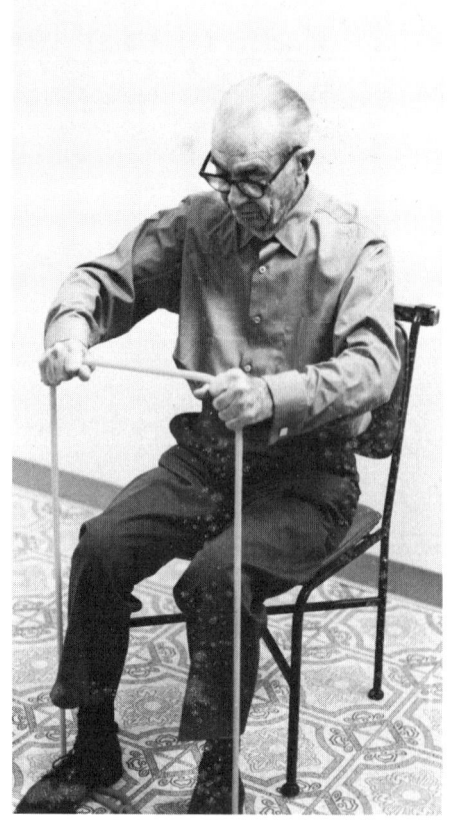

Fig. 45.

45.
Put the tubing under both feet. Grasp tubing with palms down and hands about six inches apart. Now pull up as far as you can without too much strain. As you become stronger, increase the distance you pull the tubing up.
Repeat ten times.
See Fig. 45.
The purpose of exercises 42-45 is to strengthen and condition upper arm, forearm and shoulder muscles and to limber and condition elbow and wrist joints and tendons.

Exercising a Paralyzed Arm
46.
Grasp the paralyzed arm with your other hand. Now SLOWLY move the paralyzed hand so the palm is down (see Fig. 46A.) and then move the paralyzed hand so the palm is up (see Fig. 46B.). You should exercise your

paralyzed arm even if there is no possibility of restoring movement to the arm.
Repeat as you're able.

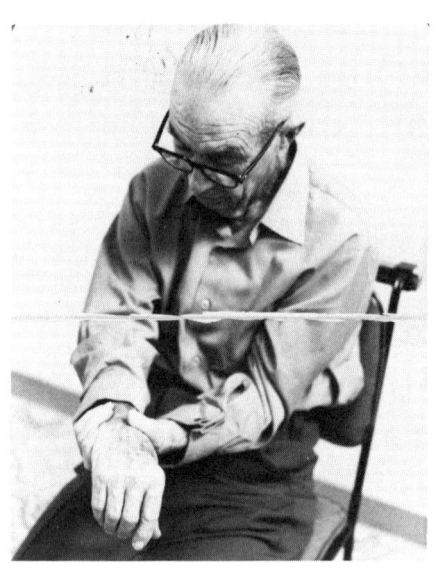

Fig. 46A.

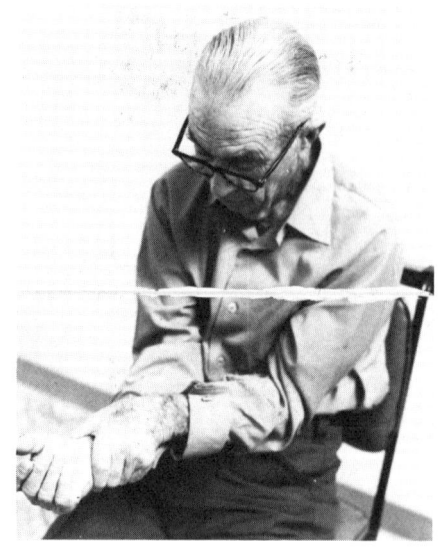

Fig. 46B.

47.

Grasp the wrist of your paralyzed arm with your other hand and SLOWLY move the hand toward the same shoulder. Touch the shoulder, if you can. Now SLOWLY return the hand to your lap. Repeat ten times.
See Fig. 47. for up position.

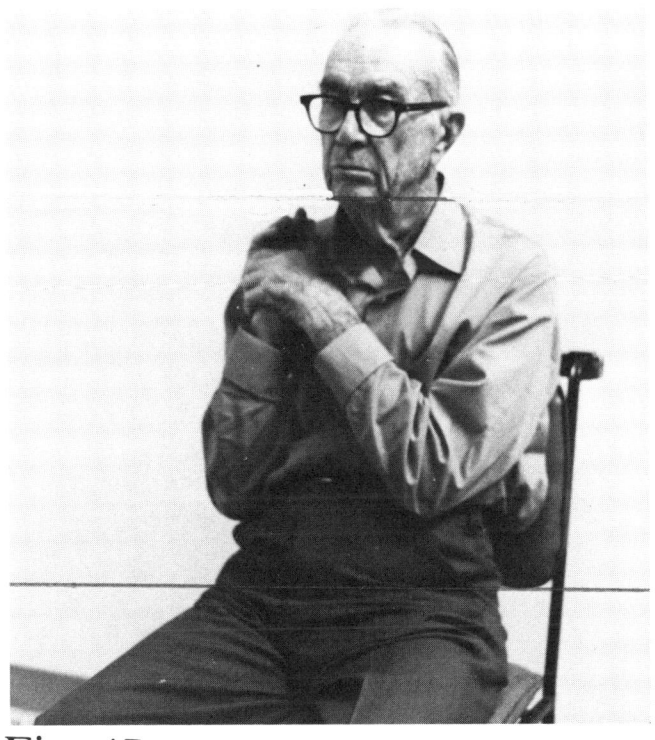

Fig. 47.

48.

Grasp the wrist of your paralyzed arm with your other hand and SLOWLY move the hand toward the opposite shoulder. If you can touch the shoulder, do so. Now SLOWLY return the hand to your lap.

Repeat ten times.

See Fig. 48. for up position.

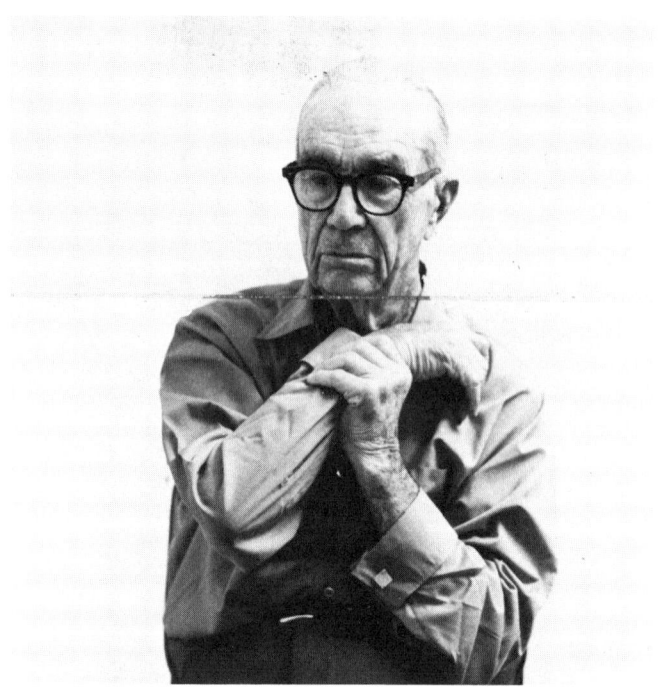

Fig. 48.

## Why Should I Exercise A Paralyzed Arm?

Even if you have no hope of ever restoring movement to a paralyzed arm, do these exercises anyway! Unless your doctor tells you not to. This movement promotes circulation to the arm. Circulation throughout the WHOLE body is necessary for general health.

## Check The Numbers
49.
Have your class hold up their hands in front of their body. Use one hand if one is paralyzed. Now call out a number between one and five. The students are to respond by holding up the number of fingers corresponding with the number called.

This checks (and exercises) the students response/reaction to a verbal command.

Do not embarrass or call attention to

those who are confused or unable to respond properly.
See Fig. 49.

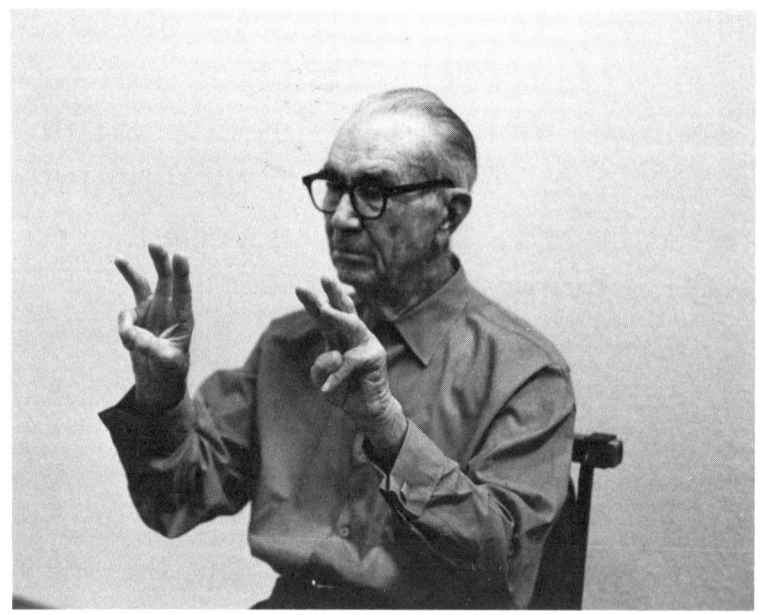

Fig. 49.

Strengthen Your Grip

These exercises can be used to strengthen your hands (grip). Certain kinds of arthritis will respond to exercise. Consult your doctor. He will advise you whether you should exercise or not. If your hands are getting weaker because you have not used them over the years then these will be excellent for you. If there are other medical reasons for a weakening condition, consult your doctor.

50.
Lay an open newspaper on a table or bed. SLOWLY crumple up one page of the newspaper until that page is all crumpled up in your hand. Continue with as many pages as you can. Repeat with your other hand.

51.
Take a cellophane wrapper from a bread bag. Open the bag and then SLOWLY crumple it up in one hand until it's just a little ball. Open the bag after each time you crumple it into a ball. Repeat five times. Do same with other hand.

# 5 Exercises For The Bedridden

I hope those of you who are bedridden didn't think we were going to forget you. This chapter is just for you. Actually, that's not true. These exercises are beneficial for everyone. However, this chapter was composed especially for those of you who can't get out of bed.
If you have any kind of heart condition consult your doctor before doing any of these exercises. In fact, if you're bedridden, you SHOULD consult your doctor first. He'll be able to tell you which you can do in your current condition.
When performing these exercises,

do not hold your breath. Try to continue to breathe normally while you exercise. I know you'll start to breathe harder because of your exertion.

## Exercise With Weights

The exercises in this section are designed to be performed with resistance. (I know, we all have a natural, built-in resistance to exercise.) That is, hold some weight in each hand when doing the exercises. You say, but I don't have any weights at home and I can't afford to buy any. O.K., but do you have two cans of soup or vegetables? A can of soup held in each hand will act as a weight and will work just fine.

If you have difficulty doing the exercises while holding some weight in your hands, do the exercises with empty hands for a month. Then do five repetitions, of each exercise, with a weight and five without. Continue increasing the number of repetitions while holding the weights until you are able to perform all the exercises in YOUR program with weights.

Don't be discouraged if you are never able to do these exercises with weights, or if it takes you a long time to reach the point where you are physically able to use them. Remember, we all work according to OUR OWN capacity. And, remember to TAKE YOUR TIME!

All of these exercises are to be performed while lying on your back.
52.
Begin with your upper arms resting on the bed and your elbows bent with your hands raised toward the ceiling. Now straighten your arms and move your hands toward the ceiling. If you are unable to straighten out your arms

completely or lock your elbows then do the best you can. Repeat ten times. This exercise is basically designed to warm-up your muscles, tendons and joints for the exercises to follow.

53.
Hold your arms straight down at your sides and on the bed. Move your arms straight up toward the ceiling and up over your head. Move your arms back down to the bed. Repeat ten times. This exercise strengthens the muscles in the front of your shoulders.

54.
Hold your arms straight out from your body with your elbows locked, or as close to locked as you're able. Form a shape like a cross. Keep your arms straight, don't bend them at the elbow, and raise them up so they are straight up in the air above your chest. Repeat ten times.
This conditions the muscles on the front of your chest.

55.
Raise your arms straight toward the ceiling, with your elbows straight. Now raise your arms even higher, lifting your shoulders up, off the mattress. Lower your shoulders. Repeat ten times.
This conditions the muscles around the shoulder blades.

56.
While lying on your back, keep your elbows bent and your upper arms straight out from your shoulders and your hands pointing toward the ceiling. Move your hands back; try to put the backs of your hands on the bed. Keep your elbows on the bed. Move your hands back to the starting position. Now move your hands in the opposite direction. Move your hands toward your feet and attempt to put your palms on the bed while keeping your upper arms in the same position.

Repeat this two position cycle ten times.

This works the muscles around the shoulder joints.

57.
Lay on your back with your arms straight down at your sides. Keep your arms straight while you move them (keep them parallel with the bed) out to the sides and then above your head. Return to the starting position. Repeat ten times.

This works the muscles on the outsides of your shoulders.

58.
While lying on your back move your hands above and behind your head until they touch the bed. Now keep your upper arms motionless while straightening your arms at the elbows and lifting your hands toward the ceiling. Return to the starting position. Repeat ten times.

This works the muscles on the back of your upper arms.

59.
Lay on your back with your arms at your sides. Keep your elbows on the bed while raising your hands toward the ceiling with: (a) Palms up, (b) Thumbs up, (c) Palms down. Repeat each of the above positions ten times.

This works the muscles on the front of your upper arms.

60.
Keep your elbows on the bed. Hold your hands up toward the ceiling. Twist your hands first in a clock-wise direction and then in a counter clock-wise direction. Twist in each direction ten times.

This works the muscles in the front and back of your forearms.

61.
Hold your arms down at your sides

while lying on the bed. Now (a) With palms down, bend your wrists up, (b) With palms up, bend your wrists up. Repeat each of the above positions ten times.

This works the muscles in the front and back of your forearms.

62.

Hold your arms down at your sides and move your wrists first to the right and then to the left.

Repeat ten times in each direction.

This works the muscles on the sides of your forearms.

# 6 Isometric Exercises

These exercises are performed by exerting effort against an immovable object (your bed) or one arm against another arm or one of your legs against the other leg. The effort put forth is no more than that of your weakest limb. So, you see, if you start out nice-and-easy, you won't hurt yourself and it's a good way to increase strength.

<u>Upper Extremities</u>

63.
Clasp your hands and intertwine your fingers in front of your chest. Firmly push your hands together. Hold for five seconds and relax. Relax for five seconds only. Repeat ten times.

This exercise conditions your front chest muscles.

64.

Clasp your hands and intertwine your fingers in front of your chest (just like Exercise Number 1.). Attempt to pull your hands apart while at the same time resisiting the motion so there is no actual motion.

Hold for five seconds and relax. Your relaxation time should not exceed five seconds.

Repeat ten times.

This exercise strengthens your back and arm muscles.

65.

With your upper arms resting on the bed, bend your elbows. Now push your elbows into the bed.

Hold for three seconds, relax three seconds and repeat.

Repeat ten times.

This exercise works the muscles on the back of your upper arms.

66.
Hold your arms down along your sides and on the bed. Push your hands into the bed. Hold for three seconds and then relax. Relax for three seconds and then repeat.
Repeat ten times.
This exercise conditions your back and arm muscles.
67.
Hold your right, clenched hand a few inches in front of your chest with the palm facing your chest and your right elbow resting against your right side. Grasp your right fist with your left hand. Now attempt to pull your right hand down, toward your feet, while resisting this motion with your left hand. Hold for three seconds and then relax. Relax for three seconds and repeat. Repeat ten times.
This exercise conditions your arm muscles.

68.
Hold your right hand in front of (above) your waist with your palm facing your head. Place your left fist in your right palm. Now try to move your right hand toward your head, attempting to bend your right elbow. Resist this attempt with your left fist so that neither hand moves. Hold for three seconds and relax. Relax for three seconds and then repeat.
Repeat ten times and reverse hands.
This exercise conditions the muscles in both arms.

69.
Make a fist with both hands. Make it as tight as possible and hold it for three seconds. Now open your hands and stretch them open fully.
Repeat ten times.
This exercise strengthens hand and forearm muscles.

Lower Extremities

70.

While lying flat on your back with your legs together and straight, push your legs toward each other. Push them together and continue pushing for three seconds, relax three seconds and repeat.

Repeat ten times.

This exercise strengthens the muscles on the inside of both legs.

71.

While lying flat on your back with your legs together and straight, push each side of your buttocks inward (the right toward the left, and so on). Hold this inward position for three seconds, relax three seconds and repeat.

Repeat ten times.

This exercise conditions your buttock muscles.

72.

While lying flat on your back with

your right leg over the left leg at the calfs, try to lift your left leg. While trying to lift your left leg push down with your right leg. Hold this action for three seconds, relax and repeat. Reverse the positions of your legs and repeat. Repeat ten times.

This exercise strengthens your hip, thigh and calf muscles.

73.

While lying on your back, put the bottom of your right foot against the top of your left foot. Now lift up with your left foot and push down with your right foot. Hold this action for three seconds, relax for three seconds and repeat. Reverse feet positions and repeat. Repeat both of the positions described above ten times.

This exercise strengthens the front and back muscles in your legs.

Some Other "Bedtime" Exercises

The following are active exercises

for your entire body. They can be performed while lying in bed.

74.
Lay flat on your back with your legs together. Now push your toes downward as far as you can. Now pull your toes up and point them toward your head as far as you are able. Take your time and really strEEEEEtch those ankle joints. Repeat cycle ten times.

This exercise is excellent for promoting good circulation throughout your legs as well as helping to prevent swelling.

75.
Lay flat on your back with your legs together; keep your legs and feet on the bed. Now circle both feet together in a large circle in a clockwise direction. After doing ten circles, move your feet counter-clockwise ten times. This exercise works the feet and leg muscles.

76.
Lay on your back with your legs straight but slightly apart. Roll your legs inward so that your toes point toward each other. Now roll your legs outward as far as you can.
Repeat this cycle ten times.
This exercise limbers internal hip muscles.
77.
Lay on your back with your legs straight. Hold your knees straight and lift your right leg up as far as you can and still be comfortable. Put your right leg back on the bed and lift your left leg as far as possible. Remember, just like all the exercises, you'll be able to move/lift your legs higher as time passes. DON'T RUSH IT!
Repeat this right/left cycle ten times.
This exercise conditions the front muscles of your hips and thighs.
78.
Lay on your back and lift your right

leg, while bending it at the knee, and move your knee toward your chest. You may use your hands to aid you in this attempt. But don't hurt yourself by pulling too hard with your hands. Put your right leg back on the bed and repeat with your left leg.
Repeat this cycle ten times.
This exercise conditions the front of your hips and the backs of your thighs.
79.
Lay on your back with your arms at your sides. Now bend your knees up and place your feet flat on the bed. Raise your head and shoulders off the bed. Reach for your knees with your hands and sit up as far as possible. Most people, regardless of age, will not be able to come all the way up to a sitting position.
Repeat ten times.
This exercise strengthens your abdominal muscles and it provides a

gentle stretching for those back muscles that tend to tighten up when a person is forced to stay in bed.

80.
Lay on your back, bend your knees and bring both feet up toward your buttocks while keeping your feet flat on the bed. Push down into the bed with your feet and shoulders and, at the same time, raise your bottom up off the bed. Imagine a rope attached to your naval pulling your stomach toward the ceiling.
Repeat ten times.
This exercise strengthens your back and buttock muscles.

# 7 Starting Your Class (professional teacher or peer group)

## Teaching A Peer Group

If you've purchased this book, began exercising and have decided to share it with someone else, congratulations. The gift of exercise is the gift of continued or improved health and enjoyment of life. It's a wonderful thing to share. I'm proud of you.

When you begin to gather a group of your friends or acquaintances together, you can be out in the open with your invitation or you can be sort of sneaky. For example, you could have a group of them over for coffee one day and when everyone is settled and complaining about aches and pains, very quietly begin one of the exercises... lifting an arm, circling a leg or something. Then, when everyone is convinced you've gone crazy, tell them about the exercise program. Ask them what they're doing to enable themselves to enjoy life better. Show them this book. It will explain to them what you are doing. Then, hopefully, some or all of them will start to exercise with you on a regular basis.

Professional Teacher

If you have just been hired to conduct an exercise class in a convalescent hospital or old age home, you will soon discover that you can't just go in and lead them in a few stretching exercises.

You will have to learn something about the people in each facility. You're going to need a versatile exercise program (in some facilities you will only use the starred exercises). You're going to need some exercise tools and you should read the paper in the morning before your classes so you can discuss current events with your group.

Once you get to your class you'll find some of your students unable to do some or all of the exercises. That's why you're there. Do not give up hope. A little exercise to begin with is more than many ever do. Work with them patiently and with warmth, humor and understanding and their general level of condition will gradually improve. Be very talkative and personable with your class. Make them feel comfortable. Make the class interesting by discussing current events, personal experiences, etc.

Starting A New Class

If you are beginning a new class and

want a gimmick to break-in the group try "Simon says". Limit the ordered movement to their arms and go slow. You'll quickly learn which students have weakened limbs, a problem with response, or a problem with co-ordination. Plus, you'll all laugh and relax together. Don't point out those who move even though "Simon says"

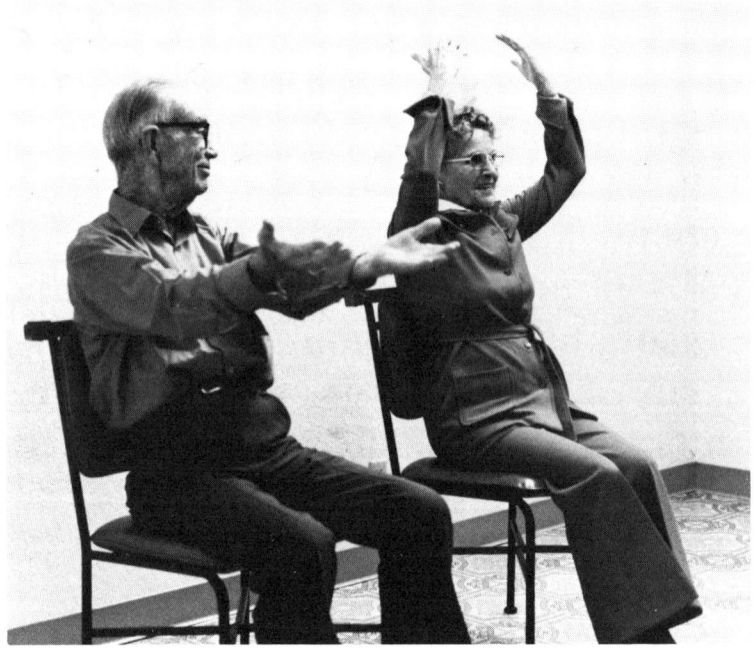

Fig. 50.

didn't preceed the command. Don't worry about winners or losers. In this class everyone is a winner just by being there. It's your responsibility to try to make them feel this way.
See Fig. 50.

Three Groups

You'll generally find your exercisers/students broken down into three basic categories:
1. Those who have had a stroke or other inhibiting physical difficulty resulting in paralysis or other injury.
2. Those who have not been exercising and are only old or out of shape, not incapacitated otherwise.
3. Those who, regardless of age, exercise in some manner regularly.

You must deal with each of these types with sincerity, consistency and specific knowledge. Even with these elements present, you'll still fail IF YOU'RE LACKING IN WARMTH AND A SENSE OF HUMOR AND UNDERSTANDING.

I say specific knowledge because you must learn what potential the various students possess. You don't want to urge a person to do an exercise which, because of a physical limitation (stroke, arthritis, paralysis) could hurt him or which he is incapable of doing. It's necessary to know the students' medical/physical problems so you know what they are capable of doing and, thus, challenge them to develop to their maximum capacity.

## For All Teachers

It's very important to remember you're not a physical therapist (unless you really are one). Your job is to provide a warm, positive, attentive atmosphere in which those who are exercising are led through a carefully chosen series of exercises. It is hoped that these exercises will, over a period of time, increase each person's endurance, range of motion, strength, interest levels, self respect and ability to care for himself.

You must give (at least try) a person hope. They'll pick up your positive attitude and eventually accept it themselves. An exercise program will accomplish all the above and more. (It might even work miracles. Though a "miracle" would probably require vitamin and mineral additives to their diet.) Check the student's medical charts at the facility or consult the person's doctor before promising anything or before providing encouragement in a specific area of performance.

Some people will, understandably, feel depressed because one or more of their limbs is non-functional. Because of this, they may have difficulty understanding the need for exercise. You must stress health for the remaining limbs, heart and lungs. I'm sure they will want to maintain and improve their current levels of activity. If not, then that's another problem you must deal with by gentle encouragement and positive suggestion and most of all understanding.

Exercise will enable most of your students to keep and improve their levels of activity. If they don't exercise they'll eventually lose additional areas of body function as atrophy sets in and morale weakens.

Provide Aids

You, as teacher, must have a few of the aids described in previous chapters with you when conducting your classes. Particularly the small loop attached to the short stick. There will always be a few students who can use these tools during the class.

You'll find some students won't exercise with the class but if you provide them with their "favorite tool" they'll at least exercise with it.

Help Combat Negativity

If you can get people re-involved in social expression through your communication and exercises, you'll find them responding more positively to all areas of their environment.

Do not just address yourself to their bodies and neglect their minds. In this way, you can provide a basis for ego building, mental and physical re-awakening and improvement. You can, then, hopefully, alleviate their two biggest enemies: boredom and depression.

Talk, Talk, Talk

Remember, exercise not only helps

the body but it helps the mind. It can lift a person out of depression and help keep him/her out of it. It can promote renewed interest in oneself and others. It can provide a foundation for a new outlook on life.

Don't just conduct the exercises and then leave. Your group will probably meet for an hour. Spend twenty to forty minutes on exercises and the rest on communication. Talk to your class before exercises, between and during exercises and after exercising. If you have read that morning's paper, then discuss current events.

When a person in your class has a very limited level of physical activity, this verbal activity can complement the physical activity for him. This added verbal exchange facilitates acclimation to the class and social interplay. And, obviously, this also encourages an increased level of mental activity.

## Open The Mind

Discuss that days newspaper articles. Learn students names, political preferences, family, hobbies, etc. Treat them as people you can learn something from. Trust me, if you're open to them and responsive, they, too, will be open and responsive with you and you will learn from them.

Don't be afraid to bring up controversial subjects like politics or capital punishment. The more you can get your students' minds working, the more they will get "into" the exercises. They will thus receive double value for the time you spend with them.

One of your most challenging responsibilities will be to re-motivate those of your students who have lost their feeling of worth and have fallen into depression.

You can begin your efforts by attempting to talk with them on current topics. After some misses, you'll learn what subjects your various students enjoy. It could be the daily crossword puzzle, sports, pollution, inflation or what have you.

This is why it is a good idea to read the paper each morning before your classes. Then converse with them as sincerely and honestly as though they were guests in your home. (Actually, you are in their home.) Don't be afraid to disagree. (Don't get in a fist fight either.) If you avoid disagreements, they will sense your fear and feel you're "babying" them and will turn you off. Their minds need challenge so don't avoid short, friendly disagreements.

Some of your students may write poetry. Find out who they are and ask them to share their work with the class. You can do this with painting, needlepoint, etc.

These suggestions can be helpful in getting your students tuned back into the real world and, hopefully, thereby developing an interest in returning to that world.

Reality Orientation

What is reality orientation? What does reality mean? What does orient mean? Reality means "that which has objective existence and is not merely an idea". Orient means to put one's self into correct position in an existing situation. In other words, this means knowing who you are, where you are and who the people are around you. Reality orientation, therefore, is a mandatory phrase in rehabilitation.

Obviously, only a few of your

students will need this type of help from you and the facility. I mention it, however, because you, with a one hour class several days a week, can present an avenue by which persons can begin to relate to their environment and themselves in an aware manner. This applies to you perhaps more than almost anyone else because your time is spent in physical activity. Physical activity which can "wake the person up" and thereby open him up to mental activity. Use only small doses at first. You should work with the facility's personnel. Discussions with them can provide valuable information about students for both of you. For example, if you notice that John Doe suddenly begins to talk after a long period of silence, make the staff aware of this so they too can follow through. In this way, they will begin to co-operate more fully with you.

## Provides A Social Setting

Exercise programs also provide a social setting. They provide an opportunity for those who are exercising to see others with similar problems working with an exercise. An opportunity to test themselves and find, often to their surprise, just how well they are able to do.

Yes, you're there for exercise but re-motivation and reality orientation are also an important aspect of your job. Your students minds and bodies are inseparable. If you deal with both, your end result for each will be far greater than if you just deal with their bodies.

This is an opportunity for communication and laughter. These are your best tools, believe me. Please use them.

## Use Of Music

Some teachers like to play music

during exercise classes. Some even develop their own tapes so the type of music corresponds with the exercise. I prefer to conduct my classes without music. I've found music makes the class less personal.

I'm always stopping in the middle of an exercise when I think of an interesting story, joke or to congratulate someone. I have conversation breaks whenever a student's behavior or comment warrants one. My students all know that they can say anything, anytime during the class. You cannot, of course, permit a total disruption of the class. This creates a sort of freewheeling atmosphere and we all feel comfortable and unpressured. It frees them to be responsive to their own thoughts and impulses or to respond to a comment by me or one of the other students. Frequently stimulating conversations have resulted.

When I've tried exercising to music I've found there wasn't as open an atmosphere for the free flow of comments and response.

I do believe that music accompanying classes composed of younger students is a valuable, fun tool.

Disruptive Persons

It's important for you to understand how to deal with a student who is disturbing the class. Some students will occasionally, or always, just sit in their chair and talk, hum or sing. If it's not too loud, then leave them alone. At least they're with other people and not stuck somewhere in a room by themselves. If they're too loud and will not quiet down, you can ask to have them removed from the class.

This action on your part serves a

dual purpose. You get the disruptive person out of the class and the remaining students learn bad behavior will not be tolerated.

If one of the students spontaneously quotes the "Gettysburg Address", "Ode To A Grecian Urn" or sings the "Star Spangled Banner" once in a while, that's another story. Let them finish, thank them for the performance and lead the class in a round of applause. They've gotten some attention and might behave for days. This can be used positively if it doesn't happen too often.

You should be reminded that most of the time a disruptive student doesn't know what he's doing so don't take it personally.

If, however, there is a student who tries to manipulate you with tears, complaints or assorted attention getters, treat him matter of factly. Be alert, of course, for a legitimate problem. Don't be cold or disinterested, just go on about the business of conducting the class. If the person becomes a disturbing factor and everything else fails, suggest that he might leave and come back another day, or have a nurse take him out. Do not let him monopolize your time. Don't be afraid to say "just a minute" or " I'm busy right now" or "wait until after class,please".

<u>Give Them Life</u>

Remember, you are dealing with people who, until recently in most cases were living full, productive lives in their own chosen environment. Modern medicine is keeping these people alive. You have the opportunity to help put LIFE in their remaining years. Years they're forced to spend away from friends, feelings of accomplishment and preferred environment.

Good luck. Your work will be rewarding.

# 8 Taking Care Of Your Back

## A Word Of Caution

Hooray, you are going to exercise, you are going to strengthen your muscles, stretch your ligaments and loosen your joints. I'm delighted...and I'M CONCERNED! Concerned about keeping you on your exercise program. Remember how I emphasized TAKING YOUR TIME in an earlier chapter? That's to avoid injuring long unused muscles and joints. There is probably a whole book on the subject of avoiding injury. Don't worry, this book's almost over. I'm just going to give you some do's and don'ts about your back.

If you take your time you should be able to develop stronger muscles, have greater flexibility and increased endurance. If you injure your back, all your hard work will not lead to any long range benefit. If, however, you take your time and take care of your back, you'll reap current and long range benefits as described in previous chapters. So TAKE CARE OF YOUR BACK.

Check Your Posture

In correct, fully erect posture, a line dropped from the ear will go through the tip of the shoulder, middle of the hip, back of the knee cap, and the front of your ankle bone. Weight should be toward your heels, your knees should be slightly bent, your pelvis tilted backward, your back flattened, your chin in and your head up.

To help you achieve this position,

pinch your buttocks together and pull in your stomach. If you maintain this position when you're standing or walking you will strengthen your

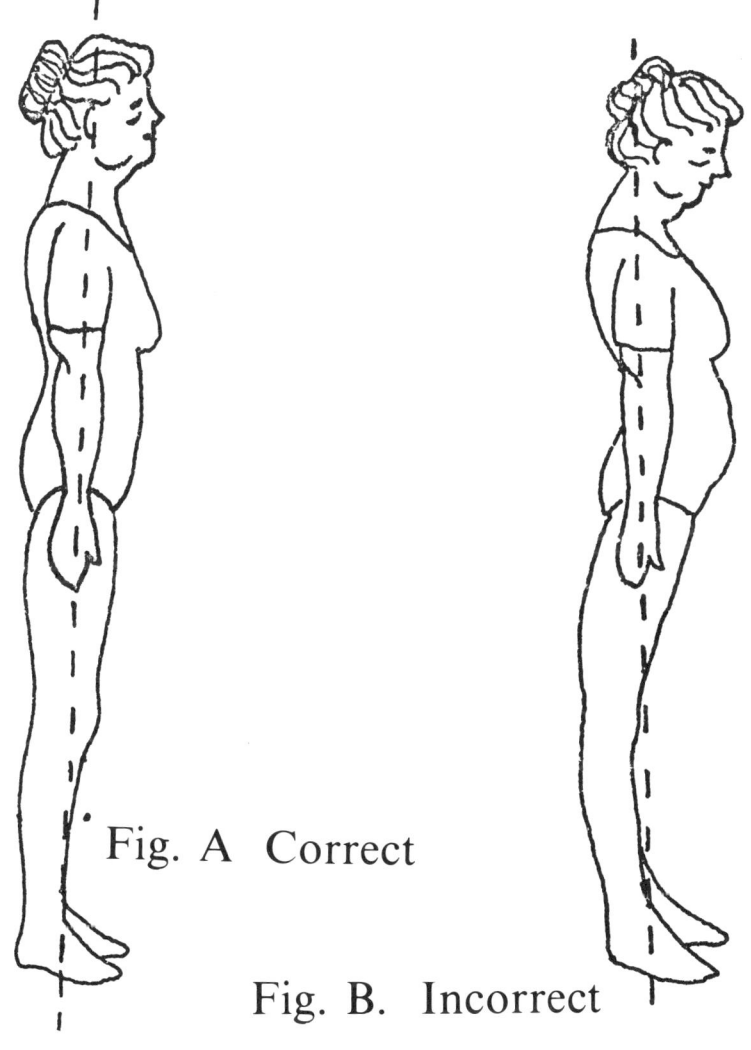

Fig. A  Correct

Fig. B.  Incorrect

main postural muscles; those are the ones which help you stand up.

## When Doing Nothing, Do It Right

Rest may be the first rule for a tired painful back. The following positions relieve pain by taking most of the pressure and weight off the back and legs.

1.
Sleeping flat on your back does not eliminate strain on the lower back. Support your knees with pillows. If your mattress is soft, place a board or piece of plywood under it.
See Fig. C.

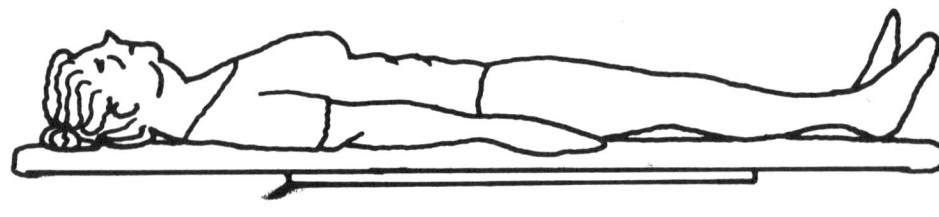

Fig. C.

2.
Use of high pillows under your head strains your neck and upper back. Do not use a pillow. If, however, you feel you must use a pillow, use a flat one. See Fig. D

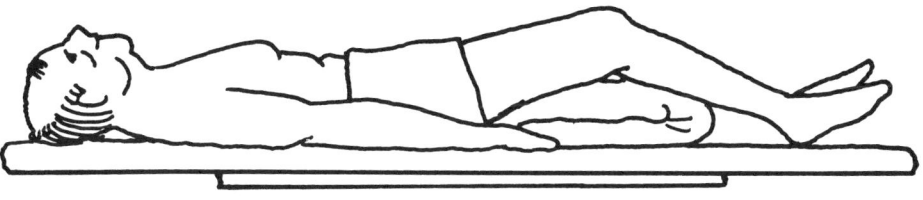

Fig. D.

3.
If you sleep on your side with your knees curled up, a pillow between your knees and your head supported, you will eliminate strain on your back. See Fig. E.

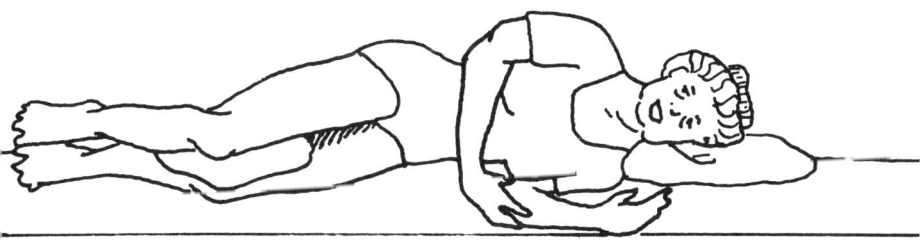

Fig. E.

4.
Sleeping on your stomach increases strain on your back. If it's necessary to sleep on your stomach, support your hips and feet with pillows.
See Fig. F.

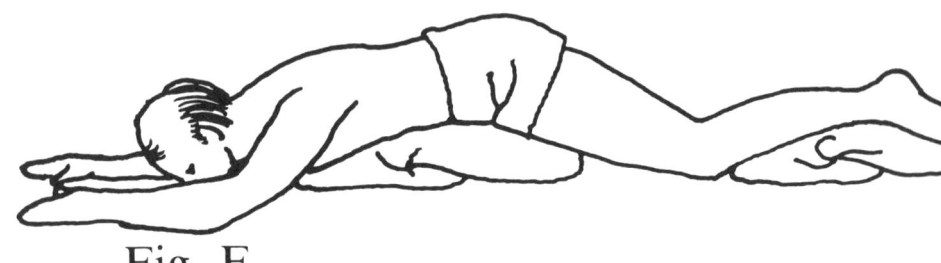

Fig. F.

5.
Here are two alternate positions to take when resting.
See Figs. G. and H.

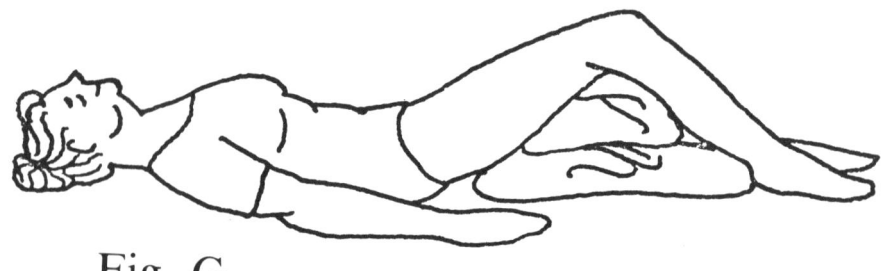

Fig. G.

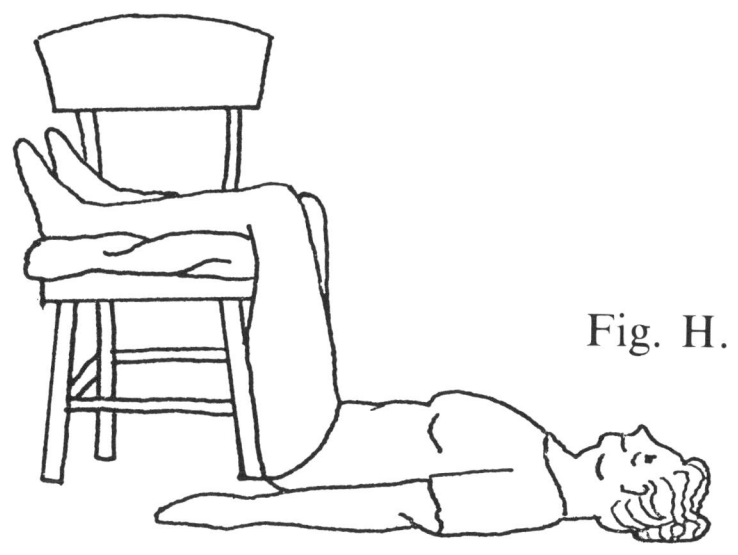

Fig. H.

Some Exercises For Your Back

There are two particularly good exercises for your back which can be performed every morning before you get up. They can also be done during the day if your back begins to stiffen up. I must point out that these exercises can be performed while lying on your bed, on the floor or even in your yard.
1.
Lay flat on your back with your legs

stretched out and together. Now tighten your buttocks, tilt your pelvis toward your head and pull in your stomach, thereby straightening and flattening your back. This relieves tension and relaxes the muscles. Hold for five seconds and relax.
Repeat five times.

2.
Lay flat on your back with your legs stretched out and together. Now bring one leg up, bend it and grasp your foreleg near your knee. Be certain you're relaxed in this position before continuing. Once you're relaxed pull your knee gently toward your chest and hold for five seconds. If you find it painful to pull past a certain point then, on subsequent repetitions, stop prior to that point. DO NOT BE BIG AND BRAVE AND "ENDURE" PAIN. I repeat, STOP BEFORE you reach the spot where the pain begins.

Repeat this exercise five times. Now perform five times with your other leg and then five times with both legs together. See Fig. I.

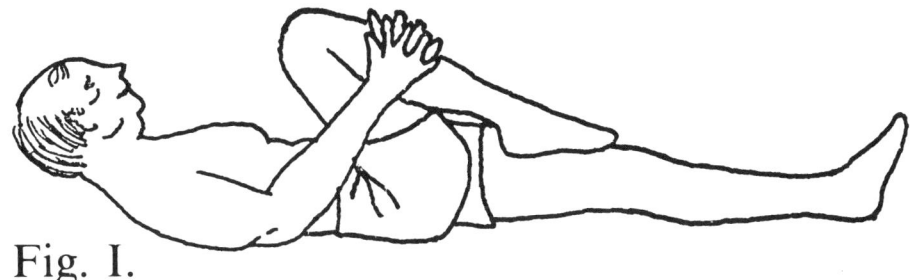

Fig. I.

### Lifting, Standing & Reaching

When picking up something bend at your hips and knees, not at your waist. See Fig. J.

Keep your back rounded as you return to standing from a squat position. See Fig. K.

When carrying something heavy hold it close to your body. See Fig. L.

Never bend over without bending your knees and tucking your buttocks under.

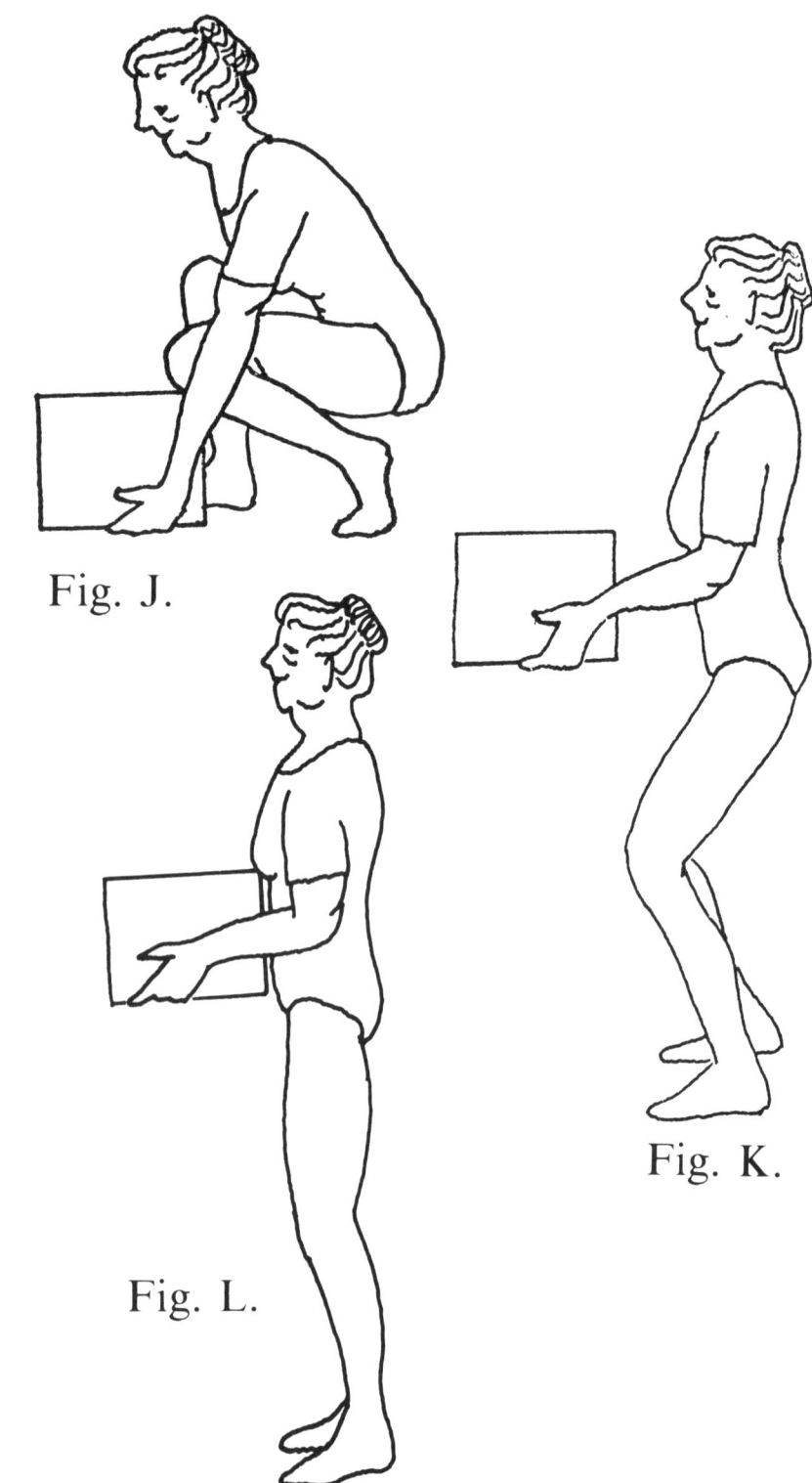

Fig. J.

Fig. K.

Fig. L.

Always face your work. When turning, pivot your feet first. When standing in one place for a long period of time, use a footrest and alternate your feet. This will relieve swayback. See Fig. M.

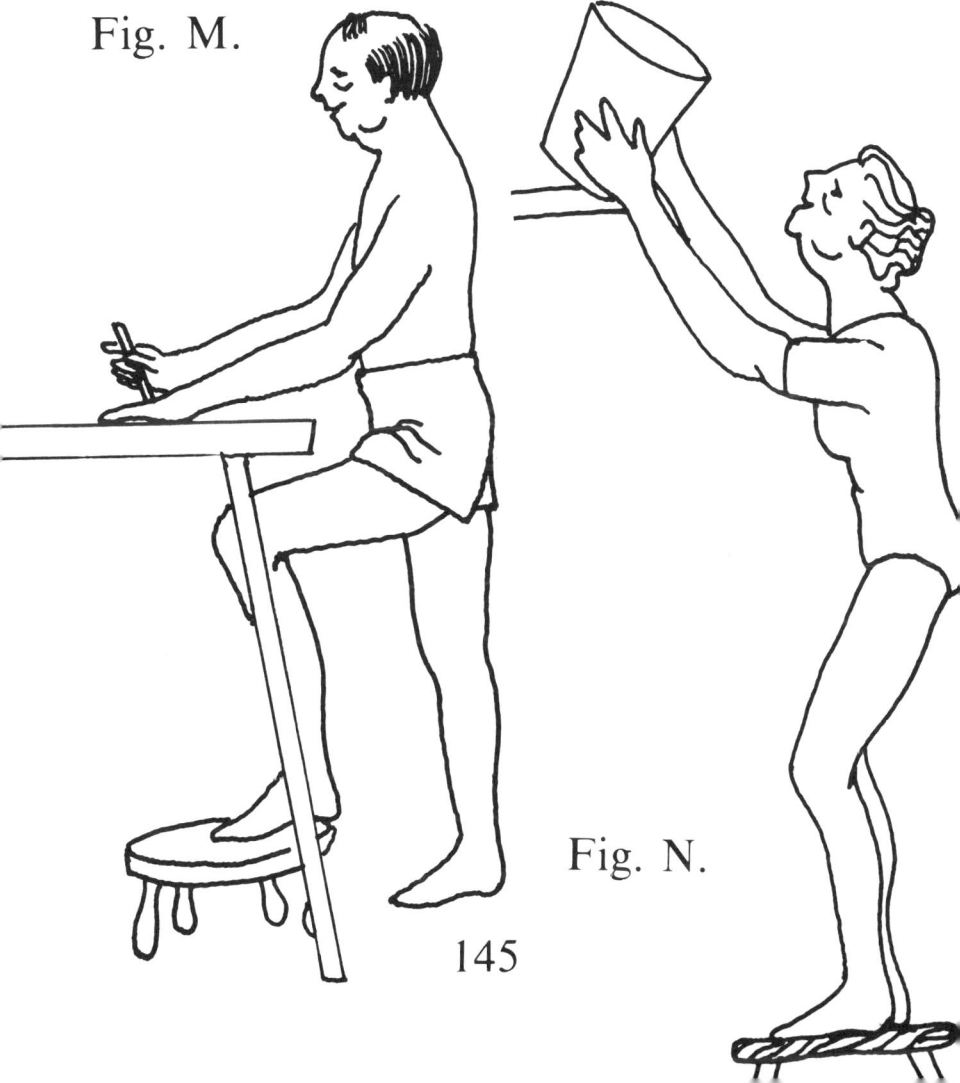

Fig. M.

Fig. N.

Keep your buttocks tucked under when you reach up. Use a stool and avoid unnecessary reaching.
See Fig. N.

## How To Get In & Out Of Bed

Starting position is shown in Fig. O. To move from the starting position to lying in bed in such a way as to avoid injury do the following: See Fig. P.
A. Bring both arms to one side.
B. Lower one side of your body to the bed while keeping your knees bent.
C. Put your feet onto the bed.
D. Remain on your side or roll into another position.

To move from a lying position back to the starting position and then on your feet, do the following:
See Fig. Q.
A. Roll to your side near the edge of the bed.

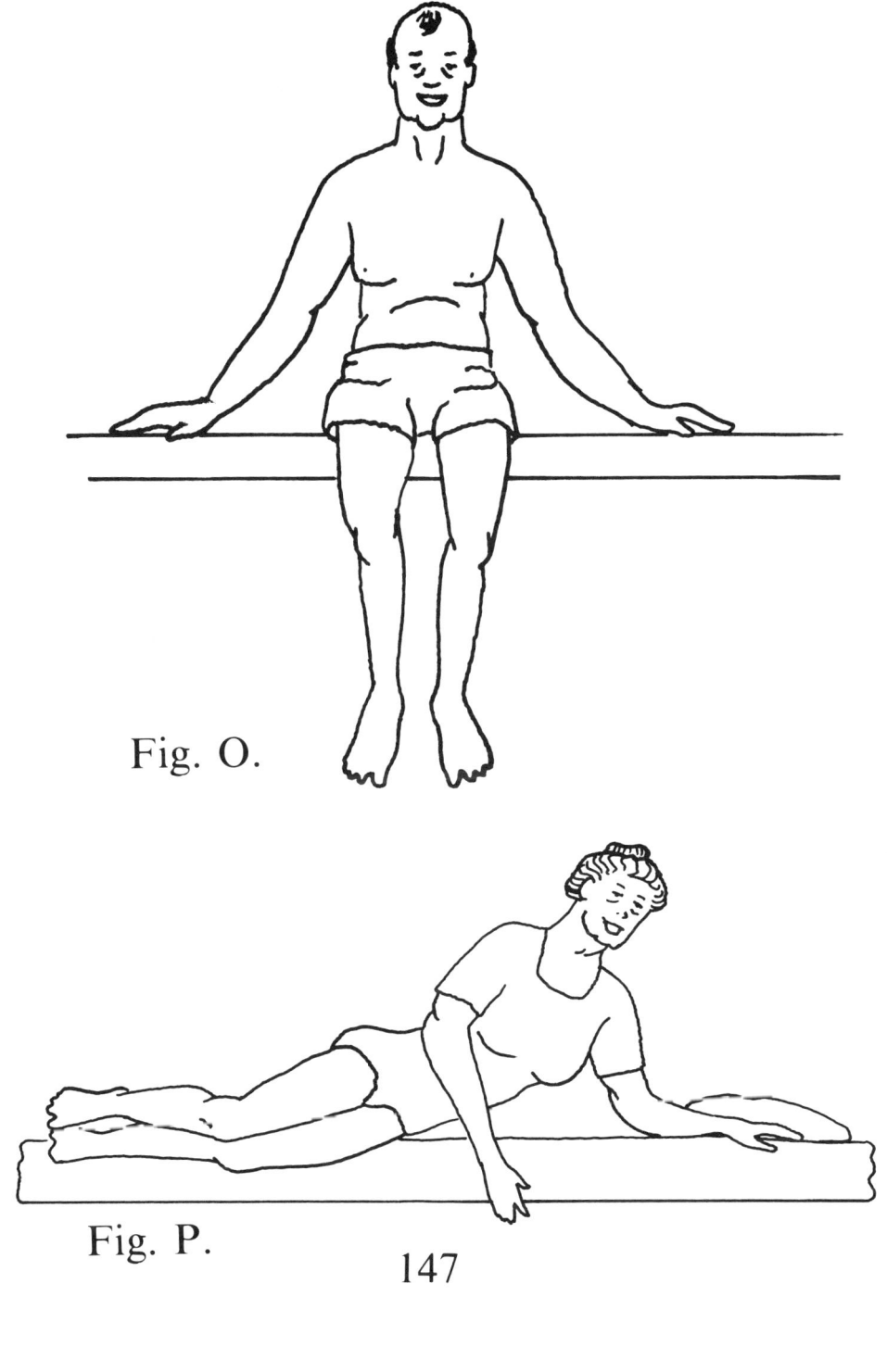

Fig. O.

Fig. P.

B. Push with your hands to move to a sitting position.

C. Now keep your knees bent and move your legs over the edge of the bed. You should now be in the starting position as shown in Fig. O.

Fig. Q.

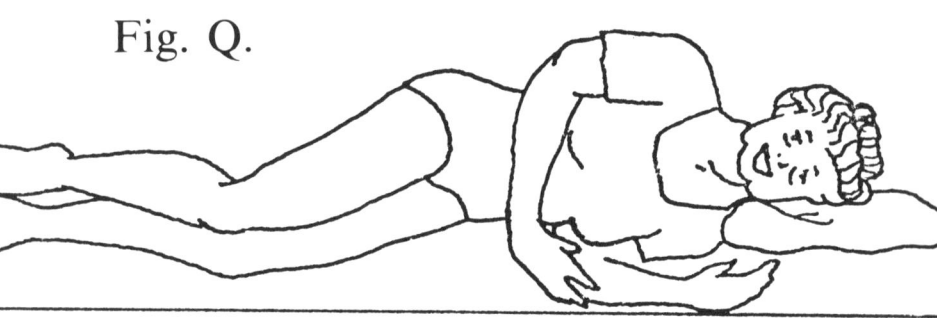

## How To Sit Correctly

Use your legs when sitting down by bending at the knees and only bending your back slightly. This is using good body mechanics. See Fig. R.

Relieve strain by sitting well forward on the chair. Flatten your back by tightening your abdominal muscles.

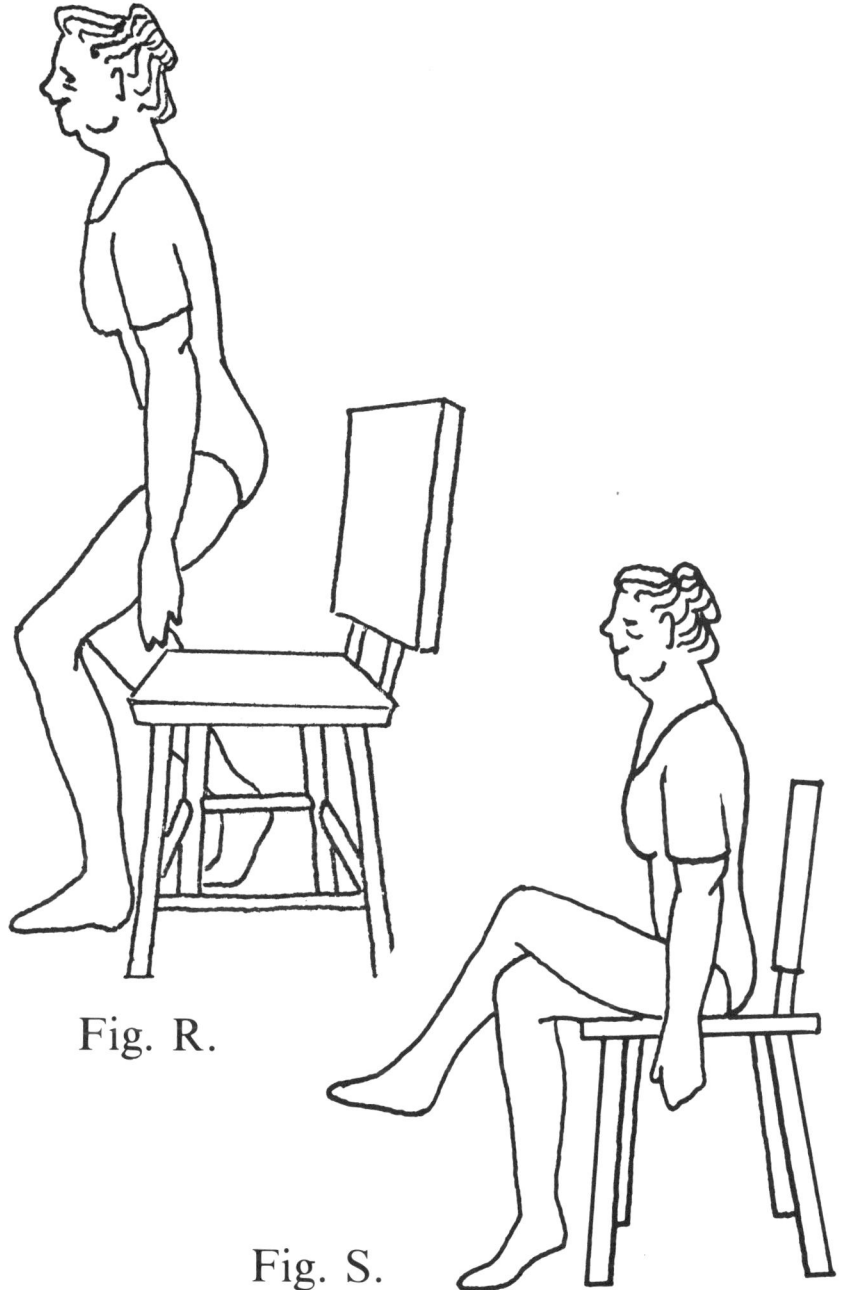

Fig. R.

Fig. S.

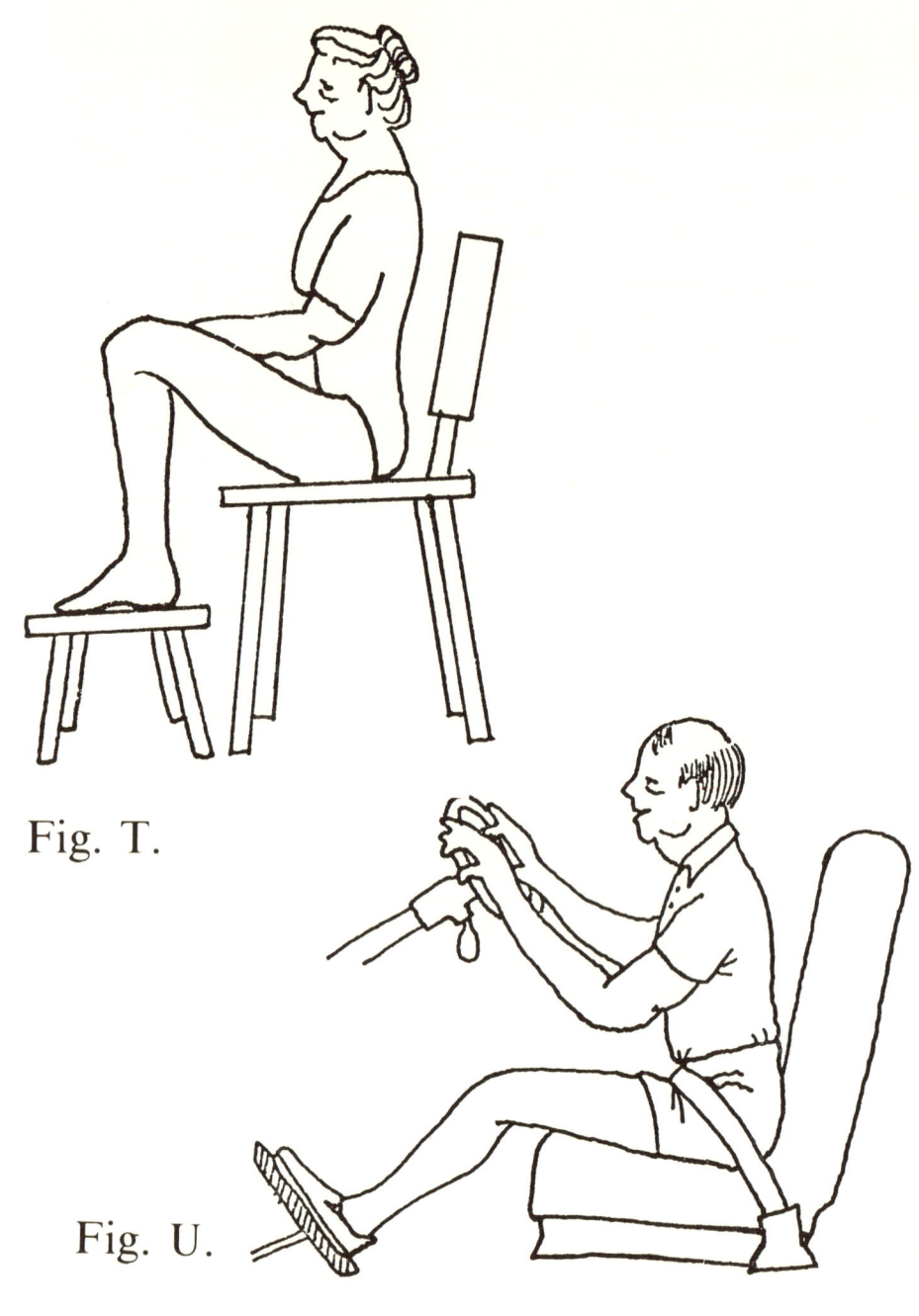

Fig. T.

Fig. U.

Cross your legs if this feels more comfortable. See Fig. S.
The use of a footrest relieves swayback. The purpose is to have your knees higher than your hips. See Fig. T. The correct way to sit while driving a car is to be as close to the pedals as is comfortable for your arms and body size. Use a seat belt and a hard backrest; this is available commercially. See Fig. U.

## To Help Ease Your Back Pain

BED

Bed rest is advisable. If you work, try to arrange rest periods during the working day. In any case, plan to spend more time in bed than you ordinarily would by retiring earlier and getting more rest on weekends.. And by all

**BOARD**

means, USE A FIRM MATTRESS!

A plywood board ($3/4''$ to $1''$ thick) should be placed between the mattress and box springs. This will help lessen the strain on your back, that is, if your mattress is not firm enough. If boards are not available at a local department store then go to a lumber yard and have one cut to order. Usually 4' × 5' or something close to that will be adequate.

**HEAT**

Moist heat is preferred. Try to relax in a hot bath for twenty minutes in the morning and again in the evening. At other times, you might apply hot towels to your back. The application of hot towels can be repeated two to four times a day if needed.

## COLD

If the use of heat does not help relieve pain, then you try cold. Many persons derive more relief from pain by the application of an ice pack. Put crushed ice in a plastic bag or commercial ice pack, wrap in a towel, and apply. Use for 10 - 15 minutes, two to four times a day.

# 9 Rules To Live By

1. For good posture, concentrate on strengthening "nature's corset" (the abdominal and buttock muscles) by incorporating the pelvic tilt into daily activities. (See "Check Your Posture" at the beginning of this chapter.)
2. When getting up from a lying position, roll to one side and push up to a sitting position.
3. Avoid all sudden movements. Learn to move more deliberately, swing your legs from your hips.
4. Avoid reaching over furniture to open and close windows.

5. Avoid reaching into high cupboards. Use a footstool.
6. Avoid lifting heavy objects, moving heavy furniture and carrying unbalanced loads which you cannot handle with ease.
7. Avoid lifting heavy objects from your car trunk.
8. Always turn and face the object you wish to lift.
9. Diaper your baby (or grandchild) by sitting next to him/her on the bed.
10. Avoid stooping and stretching to hang your wash. Raise your clothes basket and lower your washline.
11. Avoid sitting in soft chairs and deep couches. During prolonged sitting cross your legs or use a footstool to rest your back; alternate your legs frequently.

12. Change your position very often. Walking, standing or lying down may be more restful than sitting.
13. When you're mopping, vacuuming, raking, hoeing, etc., always work with the tool close to your body. Never use a "giant" step and/or a long reach in these and similar activities.
14. Sit down when putting on your shoes, socks or hose. Do not bend from the waist while trying to balance on one foot.
15. When you're taking a long trip in your car, rest your back by stopping occasionally and taking a short walk.
16. When you cough or sneeze, round your back, bend your knees slightly and contract (pull in) your buttocks slightly.
17. Avoid straining when having a bowel movement.

18. Avoid exercise and activities which arch or strain your back, i.e., bending backwards.
19. Learn to keep your head in line with your spine when you're standing, sitting or lying in bed. (See the figures at the beginning of this chapter which show correct and incorrect posture.)
20. Remember, your doctor is THE ONLY ONE who can determine when low back pain is due to faulty posture (or something else). He/she is the best judge of when you may do general exercises for physical fitness or when you may participate in a particular sport.

GOOD LUCK AND TAKE YOUR TIME!